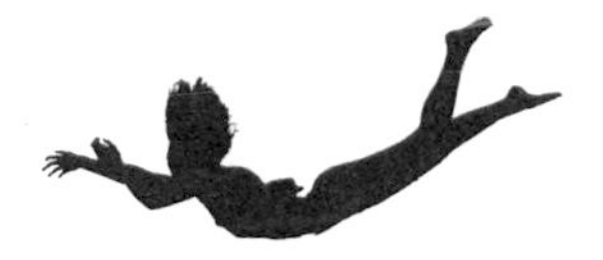

Lydia Slaby

LYDIA SLABY

WAIT, IT GETS WORSE

LOVE, DEATH, AND MY TRANSFORMATION FROM CONTROL FREAK TO HUMAN BEING

AUSTIN NEW YORK

This book is memoir. It reflects the author's present recollections of experiences over time. Some names and characteristics have been changed, some events have been compressed, and some dialogue has been recreated.

Published by Disruption Books
Austin, TX, and New York, NY
www.disruptionbooks.com

Distributed by Disruption Books

For ordering information or special discounts for bulk purchases, please contact Disruption Books at info@disruptionbooks.com.

Cover and text design by Brian Phillips Design.

Print ISBN: 978-1-63331-028-5
eBook ISBN: 978-1-63331-029-2

First Edition

TO MICHAEL,

always and forever.

May the Lord keep you in His hand and
never close His fist too tight.

—IRISH BLESSING

. . .

Every act of creation is first of all
an act of destruction.

—PABLO PICASSO

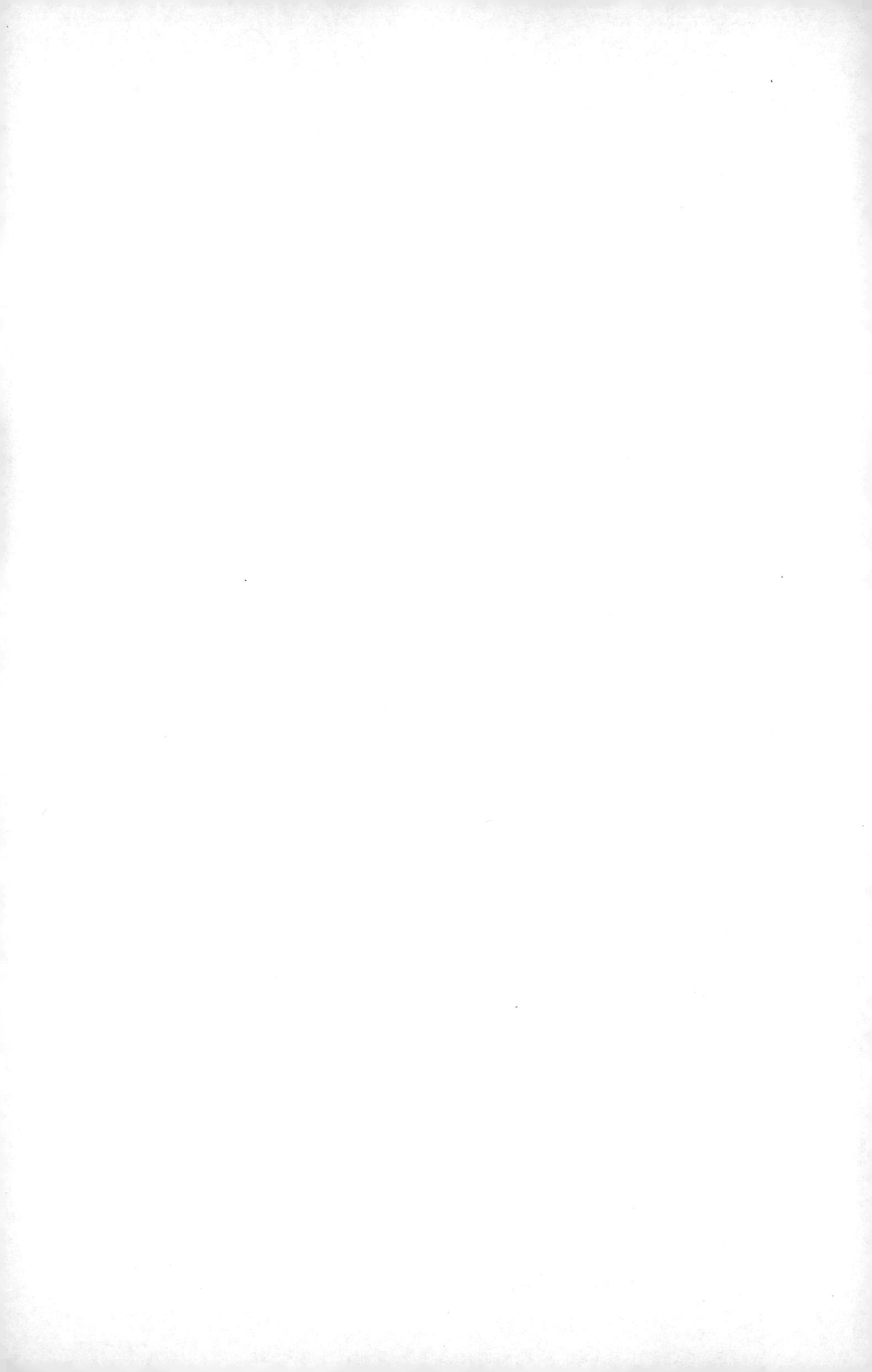

HOPE

PREFACE

THE CITY OF CHICAGO is tearing up my street, fifteen feet below my window, with massive pieces of machinery, jackhammers, and a dump truck. Even with my windows closed, the sound of crashing concrete is overwhelming, and I have work to do. Before I got sick and spent the better part of two years in and out of the hospital, I would have walked out to the men jack-hammering away and politely asked them when they would be finished with the noise. Well, I would've been *somewhat* polite. Actually, even *somewhat* is a bit of a stretch. Because when life is not going completely as planned, a control freak's reaction is to change life, not the plan.

And I'm definitely a control freak by nature.

The idea that humans can control their lives is an illusion that, prior to cancer, I chose to embrace. For much of my life, this idea helped me avoid most of the tough *why* questions: *Why am I working so hard? Why do I feel guilty all the time? Why am I the only person I know who gets bronchitis every October?*

Control freaks assume they have all the answers, and if they don't, they fake it until they make it. If I don't work hard, I won't be partner/CEO/in power by the time I'm forty! I have no idea why I feel guilty all the time, so I'll just ignore it! It doesn't matter why I'm sick! I'll just take some antibiotics, a pile of vitamin C, and do some strength training. If I'm stronger, then my body will be able to handle the bugs.

I spent the first thirty-three years of my life inhabiting this control, and it gave me two professional degrees, a husband on the verge of leaving me, and a life-threatening disease.

Changing my perspective on control did not require a dramatic change in my circumstances. I did not move to a horse farm, take off on a months-long trek, or become a yoga/surf instructor in Mexico. Don't get me wrong, I love travel memoirs—*Eat, Pray, Love* and *Wild* are two of my favorites. But I closed each book and wondered what happened when they got home and had to buy toilet paper after being stuck in traffic all day. Did they stay all zen, or did they lose it?

What did life look like *after* the transformation?

I believe the ability to *change in place* cannot be underestimated. To begin with, it was hard, even impossible, to travel extensively when I was sick, much less contemplate moving to a different city or country. But more importantly, even though traveling to different cultures always provides a learning experience, moving for the sake of moving—without taking the time and doing the work to solve the discomfort around the process of changing my perspective—would have been a waste of my time. So I stayed in my house and my city and slogged through the work of acceptance on familiar turf.

And in my case, the work was surviving—and surpassing —cancer.

This is a cancer memoir that is about more than a diagnosis and a recovery. Cancer is humbling. It's uncontrollable—even the medicines used to battle it are uncontrollable. It rarely provides clear answers to all the problems it reveals. As a result, it fundamentally changes the patient, with or without that person's permission. Cancer opens a door to transformation and makes it virtually impossible to stand still and refuse to accept the change that is happening.

Nonetheless, walking through that door is a choice. I chose at first to stand still, holding on to the door jamb like an earthquake victim. Then, after a while (here's the dramatic part), I didn't.

This is a love story. My husband and I have battled each other and ourselves for more than twenty-two years. Much of our conflict has involved accepting the reality of life with each other—sometimes this has meant recognizing life for what it is and is not, and sometimes this has meant accepting changes that each of us has undergone. Yet somehow, we love and respect each other more now than we ever did.

This is a story of integration. I learned how fundamental it is to my health that I understand my body, my mind, and my spirit as three distinct pieces of what make me a complete human being. Each piece has a role to play and a voice to be heard, and they must work in synchronicity for me to be healthy. This is a hard lesson to learn and to remember. I'm still learning it.

This is also a story of acceptance. I had to learn that *surrender* is not always a bad word. In life, there are moments—many, many more moments than we recovering control freaks care to acknowledge—when the best route forward is simply to submit to life's circumstances and see what happens.

Finally, this is my story of learning to give myself permission to be in perpetual renewal. This doesn't mean that who I am at my core changes with the wind. I am, and remain, the person who has developed over nearly forty years of life. The skills I've acquired and the history I've lived do not change. However, over the course of my life, I created stories about that collection of facts about myself, putting them into categories such as "strength" and "weakness," and then I built a personality around those stories. The power of the human mind is such that I started believing these stories with such fervor that, in many ways, I believed they were incontrovertible facts.

With the onslaught of all my health challenges, I had the opportunity to shift my perspective. My stories lost their ossification, and my sense of myself began to stretch. Some of my weaknesses changed to strengths. Some of my proudest moments became regrets. These changes in how I constructed my own stories allowed me to start reevaluating my past, forgiving myself for some of my decisions, and giving myself permission to change.

This is my story about changing my whole life, but that change is not complete. It won't be until I'm dead and gone. My life is now a work in progress—a work about finding grace, stillness, and calm inside myself, no matter the circumstances.

I wrote this book at first because I needed it for my own sanity as I sought healing and closure. And then I realized that writing it was really about how to find peace inside involuntary transitions, no matter what sparks the change, and it occurred to me: this skill might be useful to other people.

If everyone who read this book were to find a little bit of hope inside the chaos of transformation, that would fulfill my deep desire. Perhaps it can provide a small recipe for how to approach life's changes with some measure of calm. What could this world look like if all of humanity stopped reaching for the past? How would things change if instead we learned from our mistakes, took a deep breath, faced reality, and got creative about our future? All it would take is a little more acceptance and a little less panic. And every now and again, a stiff bourbon.

June 2018

DIAGNOSIS

THE FIRST OBAMACARE DECISION came down from the US Supreme Court on the morning of Thursday, June 28, 2012. Even though I was overwhelmed with editing and tracking multiple documents in my own legal case, I printed out all forty-seven pages of the slip opinion and kept it front and center on my desk, waiting for a calm few minutes to read it. My friend Gene noticed it sitting there during our morning coffee catch-up: a white stack of paper on a shiny desk on the twenty-sixth floor of a high-rise in Chicago's Loop, which housed the white-shoe law firm that employed me as a first-year associate in its corporate restructuring group.

Gene pointed to it, chuckling. "Are the gods of commerce going to let you get your fix, Lydia?"

"Probably not," I smiled ruefully, "but I'm hoping to read it on the plane to New York tomorrow." My husband, Michael, and I were heading to a friend's black-tie wedding. I had never been to a black-tie Manhattan wedding before, and I would be damned if a case I couldn't care less about was going to stop me.

"So you're still going? I thought this case had swallowed up about ten people." He sounded wistful, probably because his own work had just hit a lull, and we all worried (unnecessarily) about making our two thousand billable hours in order to be eligible for a bonus.

"It has," I confirmed, "but if everything blows up, I can bail on the rehearsal dinner and just head to the Midtown office and stay there until the service on Saturday."

I'd spent weeks plotting out the perfect dresses for both Friday and Saturday. I had lost a lot of weight in the past few months and was excited to show it off. My waist-length chestnut hair fell in shiny waves over my shoulders, a result of some ridiculous treatment I'd done the week before in preparation. An email was waiting in my inbox from a jewelry-dealer friend based out of New York with some ideas for me to borrow. I was planning on getting my nails done during lunch.

"You *are* seeing your doctor before you leave, right?" Gene's kind face wrinkled with concern. Yesterday, after jogging across the street to grab lunch together, I'd had to stop for a moment to catch my breath.

I waved him away, already turning back to my computer. "Yes, of course. I see her at eleven."

Gene laughed as he walked out the door. "Between your doctor and this case, the odds of you actually attending this wedding aren't great. Probably the same as you finding the time to do meaningful pro bono work this year."

I laughed quietly, fully aware that my personal interests did not exactly line up with my job. My work took up ten to fourteen hours a day, leaving little time for much else. But I was unsure how to make a change—or even if I wanted to. The law firm was giving me so much: experience, training, good friends, an outlandish paycheck. I was delighted with my ability to succeed in such a difficult, demanding environment. There were moments when I loved my work—the writing, the challenge, the way my mind connected dots that others couldn't see. I loved the feeling of accomplishment that came from a job well done.

But I knew my work was eating away at a part of me that I cherished. I had no time to think. I practically had no time to breathe. I felt weighed down by stress, with only the forty minutes I stole each day to walk to and from work in the balmy Chicago summer as a respite from my own thoughts.

I felt ambivalent and swamped.

I glanced at the stack of paper that I desperately wanted to read. I knew the Supreme Court had left Obamacare intact, which was a huge win for the legislation, but I wanted to see how constitutional law had changed in the process. ConLaw was one of my favorite classes in law school (honestly, it's most people's favorite class in law school), but because there are only about fifty lawyers in the United States who spend all of their time arguing issues of constitutional jurisprudence, the rest of us have to do something else. I love the Constitution—love that it actually works (most of the time), that we still live by this four-page document that declared our society would be guided only by the rule of law, a fairly simple organizational structure, and a set of human rights. But every time the Supreme Court interprets that simple document, the tides shift toward progress, away from progress, parallel to progress. I like knowing what is going on.

Oh well, I thought, turning back to my corporate case and the never-ending edits to the 150-page, legally required document that nobody would ever read. I had only a couple of hours before my doctor's appointment to finish them. *I'll read it later.*

LATER TURNED INTO *ten hours later*. And instead of being on the plane, I was in the emergency room.

At my appointment that morning, my personal doctor had detected something "off" about my heartbeat. She had held me hostage until a cardiologist at the hospital could see me later that afternoon. At the news that something was wrong with my heart, Michael had walked out of his senior staff meeting at the Obama 2012 reelection campaign and sat with me while I waited. The cardiologist gave me an echocardiogram, which showed dangerous levels of fluid encasing my heart, and had unceremoniously dumped me in the ER. It was too late in the day, he explained, for him to admit me to the hospital.

Checking into a teaching hospital's emergency room with "weird" symptoms immediately made me an interesting case—in all the wrong ways. I was not a gunshot victim. I hadn't broken my leg. I wasn't vomiting from food poisoning. My reason for being in the ER wasn't obvious in any way. I was a perfectly healthy, athletic, thirty-three-year-old, married, childless attorney, quietly dealing with the guilt of my health distracting both my husband and I from our jobs and our lives. Except now I was also an acute cardiac patient with a swollen face.

I was unable to lie down without losing my breath. So as I sat with my legs crossed on the hospital bed in my three-walled nook, with a curtain separating me from the chaos of an urban hospital on a Thursday night, the requests began.

First request: insert an IV. This is usually not a big deal, and it wasn't that night either. Except that about five minutes after they slid the needle and tubing into a vein on my left forearm, my left arm swelled up like a sausage.

"Hey," I said, waving my left arm in the air like a windsock, "did anyone notice what just happened?"

Michael looked at my arm. A nurse did the same, and then walked out to get a doctor.

"What the fuck?" I whispered to the room, which only pinged back at me in response. I was connected to an EKG monitoring my heartbeat, which was simultaneously soothing (my heart continued to work) and alarming (the pings were not rhythmical).

We were quiet as we waited for the doctor, but the ER was not. Someone next door was demanding painkillers so insistently that the nurses had called security. Outside my nook, someone else was moaning pitifully. Soft shoes were in perpetual motion past the curtain-door, moving from one patient to the next. Quiet murmuring, cries of pain and anger, shouted instructions, the occasional crash as something was thrown against a wall or the floor. . . . It sounded like complete chaos.

Yet somehow, in this place dedicated to healing, the noises were managed, held inside a container of organization that kept them away from the edge of panic. It was calm chaos, which meant people were fighting for their lives. They were being cared for by those who were trained to help. Full-blown panic—or even silence—would have been immeasurably worse to my own mind, already vacillating between the two.

Second request (as the attending walked into the room and saw my arm): "Let's X-ray your chest, shall we?"

I looked at her blankly, defiantly. "But it's my arm that's swollen, not my chest."

"Everything's connected," she responded, arms crossed, recognizing a patient who wouldn't simply comply.

"But I had an echocardiogram earlier with the cardiologist." I was confused, frightened, and tired of being poked and scanned. "Didn't they see my chest then?"

"No, they only saw your heart, which is clearly in distress. I'd like to see if there's anything there that would be causing that distress." Her face remained neutral.

Michael squeezed my leg in reassurance.

I persisted. "But the cardiologist said it was probably viral or immune-related."

"It could be. But humor me, will you?" She cracked a small smile. "I don't often to get to flex my diagnosis muscles. You have something wrong with your heart; I'd like to be thorough and see what else is in your chest."

I looked at Michael.

He looked back at me and shrugged. "Makes sense to me."

Acknowledging the majority rule, I submitted. "Okay, let's do it."

Michael peeked out into the main room as I moved from the bed to the wheelchair. With the state of my heart fluid, I was not allowed to walk anywhere. Before I wheeled past him, he gently squeezed my shoulder and said, "There's a guy covered in blood, lying on a gurney two feet from your curtain. You may want to close your eyes until you get to X-ray."

I smiled weakly. "Thanks, bear."

I kept my eyes open. The man's head was wrapped in a blood-soaked bandage, and the sheet covering his body from the chest down was spattered with blood. He looked at me through heavy-lidded eyes, and I looked back. Neither of us was in particularly enviable circumstances. Yet in that moment, blood and broken bones seemed easier to understand, if not fix, than whatever was going on with my magical arm. A fleeting thought wished we could trade places.

I stood up for the X-ray machine. First picture: stand facing away from the tubes, hugging the thick, white-screen contraption. This hurt. A lot. My breathing came in shorter, faster bursts, and I flailed about in my mind, seeking a way to relax. A tech had removed the EKG monitor and the sticky dots from my chest so she could get a clear picture. But with the increased pain from raising my arms and stretching my chest laterally, panic took the reins. I was having a heart attack, and no one would know until I collapsed on the linoleum tile floor.

Deep breath. Clear your mind. Deep breath. Clear your mind.

My meditation mantra floated through my mind like a huge banner in the wake of a small plane. Several days prior to this unexpected bout of medical tourism, I had decided to learn transcendental meditation, and I had completed the training just that morning. My older sister, Corinna, had been going on and on about it for years, having discovered it during her battle with Hodgkin's lymphoma. She had amped up her lobbying efforts in the past few months as Big Law demanded more and more of my time, energy, focus, and emotions. Finally, I had given it a try, and for twenty minutes, twice a day, my brain was quiet.

If now wasn't the moment for meditation, then I didn't know when was.

"Great," the tech said, interrupting my focus. "Now turn ninety degrees to your left, and hold on to that bar just above your head."

"Can I drop my arms for a minute? I'm having a hard time catching my breath."

"Sure, take your time."

"Um, I'm not having a heart attack, am I?"

"Not that I can tell."

"Okay." *Great, thanks. In . . . out . . . in . . . out . . .*

She restuck the monitor stickers all over my chest and upper arms, attached the wires that led from the palm-sized monitor back to the stickers, and placed the little monitor into the left breast pocket of my mint-green hospital gown. Then she wheeled me back to my nook.

Michael was sitting on the bed, scanning his phone. "Elizabeth is in the waiting room with takeout food. Mexican. Want some? Want to see her?"

I immediately welcomed the distraction from whatever medical request was coming next. Michael and I had been planning on having dinner with our friend that night. At some point, he had texted her about the bizarre and unexpected circumstances, and instead of heading home with takeout, she had brought it to us.

"Sounds great."

Elizabeth came into my nook with a quesadilla and had no idea what to do other than crack jokes and scout the doctor population for potential husbands. She was a perfect distraction.

The attending came back in. Third request: "Because of the

shadow we saw on your X-ray, we want to give you a CT scan to take a closer look."

Jokes stopped. Michael stared at the doctor. Deflated and scared, I didn't have any more defiant questions in me.

This time, they didn't transfer me to a wheelchair; they wheeled me out from the nook, right on the gurney. In the CT scan room, they didn't ask me to move from one gurney to the bed-like part of the machine. Instead, two larger men gripped the sheet I was sitting on and transferred me.

The manhandling offended the part of me that has always had a strong body that worked. "Guys! This seems dramatic. I can still walk."

They smiled and said nothing.

The tech took over. Together, we navigated the fact that I couldn't lie fully horizontal without gasping for breath in a machine that requires the patient to be fully horizontal and perfectly still. Throughout the scan, she left my heart monitor attached.

The hulking gentlemen transferred me back to my gurney and wheeled me back to Michael. And then we waited again.

The Obamacare decision was sitting on my lap, a last-minute scoop off my desk. I glanced at it off and on, trying to distract myself from the day that was unfolding like none I'd ever had or wanted. My eyes hopped across the page, skipping from word to word, my mind trying to make sense of it in order to avoid fixating on my body.

"Here's the part that the press was commenting on, about the Commerce Clause," I said to the room.

Michael and Elizabeth stopped their quiet conversation. "Oh, really?" Michael said, leaning over.

"Justice Roberts is constricting 'commerce' to only commercial activity, which in some respects makes sense, but I wonder how many civil rights issues use commerce as a basis for federal intervention."

"Wouldn't civil rights fall under equal protection?" Michael had "attended" enough of my Constitutional Law classes over Skype (unbeknownst to my professor) that we could have conversations like this.

"Sure," I replied, "but finding more than one place in the Constitution to back up a civil rights argument is never a bad idea."

"Fair point." He kept reading over my shoulder. I leaned in to his cheek, and we breathed in unison as we read.

One of the residents walked in. "We looked at your CT scan and want to talk to you about it."

"Alright." Finally, an answer!

The resident looked at Elizabeth. "Would you like your friend to stay?"

I looked at Elizabeth and shrugged. "Why not?"

The resident took a deep breath and mustered the limited gravitas that her one year of training provided her. "Well, we're pretty sure that you have some kind of lymphoma."

My brain cramped. The rest of my muscles locked into place. My vision blurred into fuzzy colors. *Huh? Lymphoma? This can't be lymphoma.*

My sister had lymphoma. Her stomach hurt, but she could breathe. I couldn't breathe, and my stomach was fine, so this couldn't be lymphoma.

When Corinna got sick a few years earlier, my parents and I educated ourselves. We got on planes and sat in infusion suites holding her hand and in hospital rooms rubbing her bald head as she managed the fallout from increasingly brutal treatments. She lost her hair, her bone strength, her muscle elasticity, her fertility, and a part of her personality. She also began to develop an extraordinary strength of spirit, which had somehow managed to become more robust following her diagnosis even when her body lacked most signs of vitality. At the moment, Corinna was living in Germany and getting a last-resort treatment not offered in the United States. Now this *lymphoma* word was pointed in my direction too, like a loaded gun.

I suddenly found myself in Michael's arms, tears wilting his starched collar. My nose nestled against his neck, breathing the only thing in the world guaranteed to calm me. My thoughts generated a picture of my sister and me, back to back with our hands extended, ready to kickbox some shadowy, amorphous killing force. "I'm never going to get pregnant," I whimpered into Michael's collarbone.

"We'll figure that out later," he murmured, stroking my back.

I turned my head toward Elizabeth. Her face was a picture of my panic.

The attending walked into the room, took one look at the situation, and frog-marched the resident out. Returning, she faced Elizabeth and asked, her voice deep with sympathy, "Is there anyone in the waiting room who you can talk to?"

Elizabeth nodded. Another friend had arrived at some point for backup.

"Why don't you go see her?" The attending steadied Elizabeth as she stood up to leave.

My EKG pinged. The patient next door plaintively begged

for pain meds, louder and louder, until the nurse threatened him with security again. The moaning out front had stopped. I wondered where my bloody friend had gone. Pinging and voices merged into white noise from the larger area just past my focus. Michael's arms were warm and secure around me, and his scent—his lovely *Michael, husband of mine* scent—kept me grounded. He kissed the top of my head and said some words to the attending. The attending responded. I nestled.

Michael started to let me go, and I squawked. "Sweetie," he said, "we need to talk to the doctor."

"You talk to the doctor. I'm going to stay right here for the rest of my life," I murmured into his neck.

I could feel his smile on the top of my head. At the same time, his hands rounded my shoulders, and we started to separate. I sighed and picked up my head.

The room was dimmer, and people had lost their crisp outlines. The background pinging was distorting into a sliding trombone of noise. The blob-shaped attending was standing near a bright screen on the left side of my bed. I turned my body around to look at whatever had captured her attention on the computer.

The pictures on the computer screen were well outside my realm of comprehension. As far as I could tell, the screen depicted a snowy landscape of alien shapes swimming in pea soup.

"Why are we looking at swimming aliens?" I asked, believing it to be a perfectly reasonable question.

The attending and Michael exchanged a look. "Honey," Michael said, "this is the CT scan of your chest cavity. The doctor is going to explain what they found." Between the *sweetie* and the *honey* and the forced serenity of his voice, a tiny part of my brain registered that he was treating me like a cornered animal.

"Oh," I responded, my voice flat. Honestly, I preferred my aliens.

The doctor spun the ball on the mouse, and the screen flashed through a series of pictures like a flip-book. She landed on one. "This picture here shows the bottom of your lungs." She pointed at two round aliens.

"Okay." My voice was still flat, but my brain was slowly turning back on, causing her face to come into sharper focus.

"These next pictures show your torso as the images move toward your head." I watched as she moved the mouse and my lungs grew. "Your heart will come into the middle, and then there's this." The picture she landed on showed my lungs flanking my heart, but there—beginning to outline my heart and occupy the remaining space between my lungs—appeared a new black blob.

The attending kept scrolling through the pictures, faster now. The black mass got bigger as my heart got smaller, and bigger still as my heart disappeared from the pictures. It faded out around the time my lungs did, at which point I could see the bones in my neck. She spun the dial again, and the pictures started moving back down my body. My mind began to formulate a 3-D model of the blob as the images flicked up and down my chest cavity. Clearly, someone had dropped a grapefruit on top of my heart and then poured molasses over the whole thing.

My heart dropped through the bed and landed with a *splat* on the floor. My palms started to sweat, and my brain went into hyperdrive. "Holy shit, what the hell is that? It's HUGE." My voice surprised me. In my head, it was squeaky and panicked and ready to bolt for the nearest escape hatch. In my ears, it sounded low and slow and calm.

"Well, that's what we believe is a lymphoma," the attending replied. "That's cancer."

My brain was moving so fast, it jammed up. I had no frame of reference for this conversation. Molasses doesn't cause cancer.

She was looking at me carefully. "Are you okay?"

My brain slowed as it registered the kindness behind her question. I had no idea how to answer. I'd spent the morning tired and swollen and not breathing well, but at work and planning on getting on a plane for a fun weekend in New York. I'd spent the afternoon being diagnosed with a severe cardiac issue, which seemed unrelated to the breathing issue. And now I had cancer.

She took a deep breath, as though gauging how much information to share, and started to explain what was going on with my body. My tumor was pushing on my heart, which reacted to protect itself by filling the sac where it lives with fluid. There was so much fluid, however, that my heart was under attack from its own protection. Every time it beat, my right ventricle collapsed. With the assault from both the tumor and the fluid, my heart was deeply unhappy.

On top of that, the tumor was strangling a huge vein attached to my heart, constricting its ability to move blood and fluid out of my upper body as it normally would. The right ventricle problem was why I was short of breath. The strangled vein was why my neck, face, and arms were swollen.

And it was getting worse. My arm had blown up like a balloon over the course of a few hours because the tumor was increasing its stranglehold on the big vein as we sat around discussing it.

Michael rubbed my hands as the gravity of the situation kept crashing over me like a series of increasingly destructive tsunamis. All day long, I kept thinking that whatever a person in a white coat was telling me right then was the worst news I was going to hear—and I kept being wrong.

"So, do I just keep expanding until I pop?" Given everything else, this seemed perfectly logical to me.

"No. Just until we figure out how to manage the tumor's growth. We're monitoring your swelling and your heart. We just need to get you admitted to the hospital so we can develop a plan for your immediate and future care."

I looked at Michael. He looked at me.

"Holy fuck," I said. "What do we do now?"

CHAOS

I WAS ADMITTED TO the hospital at some point later that night. I think it was at least two o'clock in the morning, but with all of my fear and fog and pain and swelling and exhaustion, I didn't really care. I'd just gone through a fairly sizable workup in the ER, but checking into a world-class hospital triggers certain protocols.

Sometime after I dozed off, a man came into my room with a basket—a literal *basket*—of vials for a blood draw. He took one look at the IV in my swollen left arm and at my gradually swelling right arm (apparently it was jealous and wanted to catch up) and said, "I'm going to give you an IV in your ankle just in case the veins in your arms collapse."

I twitched and woke up straightaway. Michael, who had nodded off in the chair next to the bed, did the same.

"Um," I said, "no, you're not. That sounds like the worst, most painful idea in history."

Michael agreed. "If the veins in her arms collapse, we have bigger problems. So why don't you draw the blood from the perfectly usable IV in her left arm, and we can discuss mitigating the swelling tomorrow morning with the doctor."

The tech stood fast. "I'd still like to give her an IV in her ankle."

"Bully for you," I mumbled.

"No," said Michael emphatically. "Try drawing the blood from her arm. If it doesn't work, then we'll talk."

The tech got the message and started on his sizeable task.

"What are all these vials for?" I asked, having counted at least fifteen.

His response was some articulation of words and letters and numbers, but because they didn't mean anything to me, I couldn't latch on to his meaning. So I fixated on the one distinct term he used that I did know. "I don't have HIV, so you don't need to run that test."

He shook his head. "We need to make sure." He was there to obey dogmatic orders.

Suddenly, I was furious. The past eighteen hours had been one event after another, none of which were under my control, and all of which were increasingly nightmarish and bordering on cruel. "You know," I started, "this is why our medical system is really expensive. Everyone giving people unnecessary tests."

The tech didn't respond.

Michael rubbed my hand. "Sweetie. Not worth it."

"Stop placating me," I grumbled. "He's not bleeding *you* dry." But my flash of anger had passed. I dozed off again before the blood draw was even complete.

IT'S IMPOSSIBLE TO get a good night's sleep in a hospital. People are continually walking in or out of your room, and it's never quiet in the hallway. Even when it gets quiet, the mattress and pillows are made of plastic, the temperature is less than ideal, and the lighting is always either too dark or too bright. That night, I drifted between sleep and terror, which was not a soothing combination. So when a troop of doctors plowed into my room at 8:45 a.m.—it felt more like 4 a.m., but I know the actual time thanks to Michael's detailed notes that he started taking that morning—I was already a bit delirious.

The doctors really knew how to start my day right. They ensured my increasing irritation, hunger, and confusion by using words like *mediastinum* and *biopsy* and *oncology* and *thoracic*. My favorite was *interventional radiology*. I kept asking when they were going to solve my swelling and the fluid around my heart and FOR GOD'S SAKE LET ME EAT, because those seemed to me like much more pressing problems. My priorities, however, were no match for the all-consuming process that surrounds lymphoma.

As the day went by and we spoke to what felt like dozens of doctors and they kept not letting me eat (because at any moment I might be required to go somewhere to do something for some procedure), I became increasingly annoyed. I was also completely unnerved about talking to my parents.

Until I was twenty-seven years old, my family didn't have any history of cancer. I mean, sure, my grandfather smoked his whole life and got lung cancer shortly before he died, but he was well over eighty. My grandmother was diagnosed with colon cancer in her nineties. I've always chalked both of those up to lifestyle and age. We Hills weren't afflicted with a genetic predisposition to much of anything, especially cancer. In fact, we're a pretty healthy bunch. My gardening grandmother lived until one hundred (a lesson in and of itself). The rest of my family is still thriving—remarkably so, given how much we love food and alcohol.

This pristine track record was brought to an end six years previously when my sister was diagnosed with Stage IV nodular sclerosing Hodgkin's lymphoma and started chemotherapy the day she turned thirty. *(Happy birthday, Corinna!)*

She still wasn't out of harm's way, and now I was scared to tell my parents what was going on with me. They were two for two on children getting cancer.

> Um, hi, Mom and Dad! You know how you just got back from Germany, visiting one daughter during her chemo? Do you want to come to Chicago to help your other daughter with hers?

> Hi, Mom and Dad! You remember how Michael and I were super excited about our friend's wedding in New York City this weekend? Well, we're not there because all of your children now have cancer. How's it going?

> Hi, Mom and Dad! Remember how you refuse to visit Chicago from late October through early May, when it resembles Siberia? Well, it's June, and you should totally come hang out in the hospital with me!

I mean, seriously.

All I remember about telling my parents later that day is that my father became very quiet, and my mother kept repeating,

"What the fuck?" after everything I said, until eventually we all burst out laughing. It helped.

I still have no memory of what happened when I broke the news to my sister. The fog around diagnosis is real. Michael's notes are the only reason I remember most of what happened those first few days.

HALFWAY THROUGH MY first afternoon as a hospital patient, I was insane with hunger and thirst. Michael paged the doctor, who came into my room a few moments later followed by a trail of residents.

"What's the delay?" my husband demanded. "She hasn't eaten since lunch yesterday. She's thirsty. She has fluid in her pericardial sac and what's possibly cancer growing in her chest, and all we've done is sit here all day. This is unacceptable. When are things going to start moving?"

"Well, you see . . ." The doctor hemmed and hawed and said something about "scheduling" and "typical Friday afternoon."

Michael's response was pointed and filled with colorful language. I watched the whole thing with the interest I usually devote to a tennis match on television (not much) and tried to ignore the sandpaper in my throat.

After Michael threw that doctor out of my room, one of the residents intervened. "The real problem is that Interventional Radiology was completely booked in advance today," he explained, "and it's hard to convince the doctors down there to stay late on a Friday."

Michael looked him straight in the eye. "I appreciate your

honesty. Thank you. But if any one of those doctors leaves for the weekend before draining Lydia's fluid or giving her a biopsy, then they better come up here in person and tell me why."

Half an hour later (time according to Michael's notes: 5:15 p.m.), I was wheeled into Interventional Radiology. We never saw the older doctor again. I began to notice that the younger doctors, the ones who were about my age, bent over backward for me. Was it because I was their age, and the whole idea of an ailing thirtysomething was scary to them? Or did they just have more energy to massage the system? Whatever the cause, if I needed something and the first doctor's answer was invariably "no," I always had better luck with someone younger.

Interventional Radiology, or IR, is where doctors do things with tiny catheters and needles while you lie very still on a table with X-ray machines and ultrasounds and all sorts of other machines pointed at you. The doctors were looking at this screen and that screen to make sure their tiny catheters and needles were going to the right spot. Nurses and techs were doing things I'd only ever seen on television shows: holding their hands up in the air to avoid touching anything, dumping sterile equipment onto sterile sheets, putting on gloves to remove a pair of gloves from packaging, replacing that set of gloves with the two new layers of gloves they'd removed from the packaging. The room was an icebox—frigid and sterile and both intensely bright (under the floodlights) and deathly dark (in the shadowy corners of the room).

The whole thing put me on edge.

My hunger was acute. My thirst was grating. I was weary and blurry, and now they were about to do something to me that required layers upon layers of sterility. Nobody had ever done anything to me that required this level of cleanliness—except possibly once, when I had my lung reinflated after an accident in New Zealand, but I don't remember the details of that day. The tools of the ER—X-rays and blood draws and stethoscopes and CT scans—I understood. Mostly. This was not that.

Just when panic was about to take over, into my life tumbled Tweedledee and Tweedledum, possibly the only two doctors the hospital could dig up who were willing to stay late on a summertime Friday afternoon for a bizarrely sick woman and her obstreperous husband. And I'm so glad they did.

One was young, a resident, and the other was older but not by much. Although they were about to do impossible work with tiny instruments on the tender area around my heart, they took it upon themselves to adopt silly caricatures simply to help calm me down. To me, this was evidence that both men were clearly talented doctors. They were the first to show me that I wasn't just a diagnosis, but a human—a real, live person with fears and feelings that needed to be addressed and treated. They saw that my emotional well-being was just as important as my physical wellness.

For the next year, these two would unexpectedly pop into my life like a jack-in-the-box, making me laugh during scary or physically painful moments. Our journey together began that night.

"So, we hear you're sick," said Tweedledee.

"That sucks," said Tweedledum.

"What we're going to do is give you two drugs, fentanyl and Versed, which will put you into a bit of a twilight state . . ."

". . . which we're sure you already feel like you're in, because of the shock of the news . . ."

". . . and we'll do a needle biopsy on this bad boy to see what we're dealing with . . ."

". . . shouldn't hurt a bit, but let us know if it does or if you're going to have a panic attack or something else that would cause you to move . . ."

". . . we really don't want you moving, because we really don't want to poke your heart..."

". . . yup, you've got enough problems . . ."

The pitter-patter of their voices went on and on, laced with humor and concern and words I could understand, and I immediately relaxed, an image of the cartoon versions of their namesakes bouncing through my head. A nurse scrubbed down my chest with Betadine, and the two doctors lined the area of the incision with sterile blue cloth. One of them told someone else to "crank the medications," and I was out.

When I next opened my eyes, I was back in the recovery area. The soft summer evening light was streaming through the window, backlighting everything around my bed. Michael was a hazy mass standing at my feet, talking to a woman I didn't recognize. They noticed that I was "awake" and turned to me.

"Hi, Lydia. I'm Rena Levi, your oncologist," said the woman. "Your primary doctor has been tracking your medical notes. She called me this afternoon and told me to come find you. I'm so sorry that we're meeting under these conditions." This apparition, pulled from my primary doctor's magic hat, was entirely lit from behind, so I couldn't tell what she looked like at all. She seemed like an angel who had just dropped out of the heavens.

"Hi," I whispered, still woozy from the drugs and shell-shocked by the realization that I now had a doctor who specialized in cancer. My heart began to open up in gratitude and awe toward this team of experts who were entirely focused on my health.

Dr. Levi came around to the side of my bed, where I could see her more clearly—tall, perhaps a little older than me, with kind eyes that held sympathy and pain. She took my hand in hers and told me everything was going to be okay. She talked about a lot of things that evening (according to Michael's notes). The only thing I truly remember is this: the tumor appeared to be of a non-Hodgkin's variety, and the medical establishment knew and understood how to battle it.

Michael softly squeezed my foot, and my eyes misted with tears.

Then Tweedledee and Tweedledum tumbled back into my room, announcing they were taking me back to IR to insert a pericardial drain ("Because having that much fluid in your heart sac is a total bitch," said one, to which the other responded, "Yes, let's get you breathing again"), and the rest of the evening faded into an opiate haze.

THE NEW YORK WEDDING was stunning. The mighty Hudson River played witness to an intimate service in the dazzling light of a June morning. The party that evening was a massive blowout with fantastic music and dancing until the wee hours.

Or so I heard.

That Saturday morning, as our friends exchanged vows and voluntarily walked over that threshold that transforms people worldwide from *me* into *we*—their future together an unwritten yet hopeful story—I was thrust into a transition of my own. A kindly gentleman wheeled my gurney through sneaky underground passages from the main hospital to the women's hospital, where (on the lower floors) babies fought to be born and (on the upper floors) cancer patients fought for their lives. He ferried me into the patients-only elevator and up to the fourteenth floor, and then rolled me into a sunny room where I would spend the next two weeks looking out over Lake Michigan. My transition took me from health to sickness, from vitality to frailty. From the self I knew to one who had yet to be formed.

It was official. I was a cancer patient.

CANCER

THE DAY BEFORE I suddenly had cancer, I sat in front of my computer until 1 a.m., hard at work on a very detailed legal document. I had exercised with a trainer the day before that (with unprecedented shortness of breath, in hindsight). But once I gave my body permission to be exactly what it was—sick and tired—I was useless.

Walking a lap around my hospital floor required a three-hour nap afterward. Yet letting my body do what it wanted to do was remarkably freeing. I found myself becoming calmer in the moments when I indulged the sheer exhaustion and let the present moment be exactly as it was. I'm sure the fatigue was partly my brain protecting itself from the onslaught of frightening information, but the bottom line is that I must have been really sick for a long time and just never acknowledged it.

My tumor was the size of a grapefruit. It had been growing for at least eight months, but most of the growth, as with the newborn babies in the maternity ward downstairs, had happened in the past couple of months. The doctors knew this not only for fancy medical reasons, but also because of the progression of my symptoms. I was generally fine until April and only started suffering from shortness of breath in mid-May, a month before my diagnosis.

The catheter installed like a plastic corkscrew near my heart drained off more than 400 cc of fluid during that first twenty-four hours, which made my doctors very happy. As the balloon of fluid emptied, however, the catheter was no longer floating in the space between my heart and the pericardial sac, and instead started rubbing up against my heart muscle. And that felt about as good as it sounds.

At the same time, Dr. Levi put me on massive doses of steroids intended to shrink the tumor enough to release that massive vein. I found out a few months later that I was "lucky" the tumor had not already caused the vein to rupture, thus bleeding me out and killing me fairly instantly. So even though I was concerned about my labored breathing and the pain from the plastic pig's tail rubbing my heart, the hospital was much more concerned about getting the growth of the tumor under control.

As my first weekend in the sunny room on the fourteenth floor turned into a Monday, my schedule of perpetual napping was interrupted by a parade of people assigned to help prepare me mentally and physically for the onslaught of chemotherapy. This included a full dental exam (chemo makes one susceptible to cavities, so it's best to start with none) followed by a bone marrow biopsy (one of the most painful procedures I've ever endured) followed by a visit from the onco-fertility specialist (a bit of a miracle given that, at the time, only two hospitals in the country even had someone specializing in fertility issues associated with cancer and chemotherapy) followed by a PET scan (an injection with radioactive material that cancer loves to eat, and then a full-body scan to determine where the cancer is active). Procedure followed procedure, ad nauseum, culminating in complete depletion.

All of these painful, invasive examinations revealed that my cancer existed only in the known tumor, which was good news, and that my body and teeth were healthy enough to start chemotherapy—once they knew what kind of cancer I had.

Lymphoma is divided into two major categories: Hodgkin's (what my sister had) and non-Hodgkin's (what it seemed I had). There are twenty-three versions of non-Hodgkin's, most of which present differently in that they grow at varying rates, arise in assorted areas of the body, appear in people of various ages, and require a range of treatments. As the experts worked on this question, I had some of my own.

"If I only have cancer in my tumor, then why don't you just cut it out and send me back to work?" I asked Dr. Levi, hoping that her vast medical training was somehow incomplete, and that she had overlooked such an obvious course of treatment.

She dealt a devastating blow to my amateur solution, explaining that because lymphoma is a systemic cancer, it could be floating around my entire lymph system. "So even though it's only presenting in your chest right now," she said, "we need to kill it systemically, which we can only do with chemotherapy. Otherwise, it will pop back up somewhere else."

I tried again. "If the steroids are doing a good job of reducing the size of the tumor"—which they seemed to be doing—"why can't I just stay on them and bail on the chemicals that will diminish my fertility?"

Dr. Levi smiled kindly. We were quickly learning that I was going to push as hard as I could to take ownership over my treatment. "Because steroids can only contain the growth of the tumor, not actually stop it from being cancer. You would have to stay on steroids for the rest of your life. And even then, you have such a fast-growing version that they probably won't work for more than a month anyway."

I soon learned that some forms of non-Hodgkin's lymphoma aren't particularly aggressive. A tumor shows up, and if it's not growing quickly, then a weekly or monthly medicine keeps it small and the patient simply lives with cancer. Of course, mine was not one of those lazy tumors, which was deeply disappointing. The prospect of chemotherapy terrified me, even as a tiny part of me was strangely proud of it. This was *my* tumor, after all. It had moved into some prime real estate, started with its natural talent, and—through dogged persistence and determination—achieved well beyond normal expectations. If you're going to do something, you might as well do it right.

By this point, a few days into my hospital stay, the steroids had kicked in. I constantly felt as though I was on a low-grade caffeine buzz. The 'roids were working well enough: my sausage arms had deflated, and I could see the tendons in my neck again. At the same time, the twice-a-day EKG was showing that my heart was "irritated," to which I commented, "It might have something to do with the piece of plastic jammed in my chest." The doctors took out the pig's tail, and my resting heart rate dropped from 80/90 to 50/60. I took my first deep breath in months.

Between being able to breathe and not feeling like my cheeks were going to explode, I found my sleep finally became restful, and I began to regain a bit of my former vigor. With renewed energy, however, I became aware that I was trapped in the hospital with cancer and no plan. I started growing antsy. I would wander off when nurses needed me, seeking refuge on the exercise bike in the visitor's lounge. Desperate to exert some kind of control over my plight, I started picking little fights about every single medication they wanted to give me. When one shot burned like hell, and I discovered it was a blood thinner to prevent clots as a result of my being too sedentary, I had my first conversation about which medications I truly needed. Considering I was having this slightly testy chat with my nurse while I was pumping away on the bike, my team agreed that I could stop having that particular shot, as long as I kept moving.

Just when I got so antsy that I decided to walk right out of the hospital, with or without my IV stand, my doctors arrived at a diagnosis: diffuse large B-cell lymphoma involving the mediastinum—stage II. It breaks down like this:

Lymphoma: Cancer involving the lymph nodes
Mediastinum: Part of the body in the middle of the chest, above the heart and between the lungs
Large B-cell: A kind of white blood cell
Diffuse: Spread out
Stage II: Not as bad as Stages III or IV, but worse than Stage I

After Michael carted the biopsy slides away to another hospital for a second opinion, Dr. Levi explained the treatment protocol: something called R-EPOCH, a combination of a new antibody drug (*R*), steroids (*P*, for prednisone), and old-school mustard-gas chemotherapy (*E*, *O*, *C*, and *H*).

The *O* and the *C*—Oncovin (aka vincristine sulfate) and cyclophosphamide—are the worst two in this pile of letters, causing side effects like vein desiccation and infertility. Because the vincristine could burn through smaller veins, it had to be administered slowly, into a very deep, thick-walled vein, and, even then, checked frequently to ensure that it hadn't burned through those walls.

To administer this cocktail safely, the doctors required me to stay in the hospital for about a week, once every three weeks (barring any complications or unforeseen visits) for at least six and possibly ten treatments. After performing some quick math, Michael and I stopped being simply courteous to the nurses and techs on my floor and started making friends.

IN THE MEANTIME, gifts were flowing into the hospital from all over the world: chocolate, books, iTunes gift cards, balloons, stuffed animals, and love. "The best part about cancer?" I exclaimed to Michael as I unwrapped a package holding slippers and sweatpants. "The fuzzy presents!"

My parents gave up on getting phone reports and just showed up on the Fourth of July to make sure that, other than the cancer, I was okay. Friends in Chicago brought takeout and played card games. Work told me not to worry about a thing, and we would sort things out once I could think straight. The extraordinary generosity from everyone I knew helped support Michael and me through everything that we were managing: all the complicated conversations with doctors about treatment options and all the physical hurdles I had to clear.

To get down to a vein deep enough for the administration of my particular cocktail, they needed to install a "central line," which is basically a permanent IV that accesses a deep vein instead of a surface vein. Until my tumor shrank enough, I had to start with a PICC line. So I went back to Interventional Radiology, where they gave me a little cut on the inside of my right bicep, found a deep vein, and shoved a foot and a half of tubing into it, which extended into my chest. Then they attached the part still waving in the breeze to a contraption that split the single tube into three, anchored the whole thing to my skin, sterilized it, and covered it with an oversized plastic bandage. This still completely grosses me out.

So I had a three-fingered plastic tube dangling from the inside of my arm that the nurses used for blood draws and drug administration. If I looked carefully, which I did only once, I could see the pencil-thick tubing going into my arm slightly pulling in and out a little every time I moved. I immediately cut the toes off a pair of socks and covered the whole thing up so I wouldn't catch it on anything or, worse, think about it. Then I kept pestering Dr. Levi about when I could get a port, which had the advantage of being entirely subcutaneous.

We also kept asking about—and Dr. Levi kept refusing to give us—mortality or morbidity statistics. "The mortality rate on your form of cancer in your age group is generally very good, but I'm not giving you numbers," she insisted. "We will give you the treatment that we know will help kill off the disease. If it doesn't work, then we'll go on to next steps." She refused to either frighten or excite me for no reason other than to satiate my curiosity. "Feel free to Google it, but I recommend that you don't."

She made similar comments about the treatment protocol. "You will lose your hair, your immune system will collapse, and you will get absolutely exhausted. But otherwise, you might experience any number of side effects from the chemo—or you might not. I'm not going to give you the complete list, because it will just freak you out. We'll deal with them as they arrive." She felt that my energy would be better spent dealing with my reality, not my fears.

Dr. Levi was right. I would either die, or I wouldn't. Therefore, the mortality statistic in my personal case was either 0 percent or 100 percent. Knowing how other people fared wouldn't change that reality one bit. The best I could do was stay focused on my own health and notify her if I felt any different from day to day. So I never researched my diagnosis.

Others did, however. The most unhelpful comment I ever received was from a particularly obtuse family member. He informed me that if the words in my diagnosis were rearranged—into a different diagnosis, I presume—then my chance of survival would be better. I hung up, sighed, and went back to watching Wimbledon on TV.

WITH R-EPOCH, I had a 5 to 10 percent chance of losing my fertility. As I discovered with the mortality rate conversation, this statistic is entirely useless. Chemo ages a woman's ovaries. This particular chemotherapy cocktail would age my ovaries by a few years. So the only way to know what that really meant would be to know when my body would begin going through menopause in the first place. Medicine hasn't solved that particular mystery, so the best I could do was ask my mom when she went through her own menopause—and then do everything I could to protect my body from the onslaught of toxic chemicals.

Like my treatment, my fertility options seemed a bit medieval. Option one was to protect my ovaries as best as possible during treatment by chemically shutting them down with drugs. Chemo attacks fast-growing cells, and an egg maturing in an ovary is, by definition, a fast-growing cell. By preventing eggs from growing, the ovary itself can shield the eggs from danger. Theoretically, anyway. Side benefit? I would lose my period. Considering I was having a hard time walking in a straight line most days, not having to deal with a monthly menses sounded like a blessing. Awful consequence? In addition to all of the side effects from chemo, I would go through the symptoms of menopause for the duration of the treatment. I learned this after the fact.

The second option was to harvest and freeze my eggs, with or without fertilizing them first with tiny Michael sperm. This seemed like an exceptionally practical option, right up until I learned the details and really thought it through: Twice daily shots that trick the ovaries into producing ten to thirty eggs. Feeling like garbage as hormones fluctuate all over the place. A vaginal ultrasound every forty-eight hours—not the kind of ultrasound featured in a heartwarming movie-moment as a wand gently glides across a woman's belly to reveal the first thrilling glimpse of her baby, but rather a cold, dildo-like device that is covered with a condom and unceremoniously stuffed up one's snatch. And then, if I'm lucky, after two or three weeks of this horribleness, they put a microscopic vacuum cleaner next to my ovaries and suck out the eggs that are mature enough to be harvested. "That part doesn't really hurt . . . much," a male doctor informed me.

If I froze them unfertilized, 4 percent might survive. If I froze them fertilized, 50 percent might survive. Michael could get hit by a bus or otherwise leave me, and then my only option for children would be miniature Michael embryos, which would then remind me of my departed husband for the rest of my life. Or all these harrowing procedures would simply yield a pile of cold, dead, single eggs. That was a fun conversation.

Option three would be to harvest an entire ovary and freeze it, and then magic happens. This option was so ludicrous that I couldn't even think it through.

Option four was to do nothing and hope for the best.

Oh, and we need an answer on this by tomorrow, so if you could just take the next twelve hours to think through all the long-term implications of possibly losing your fertility and all the ways we can try to make sure you can have children (if you even decide you want to someday), that would be great, thanks.

"So, if I decide to harvest my eggs, you'll delay chemo by a month or something?" I asked Dr. Levi. As with my questions around chemo, I believed this was an entirely appropriate solution to my predicament.

She responded kindly but firmly. "No, you're in an emergency situation with your tumor, and we would be shirking our medical duties if we let you delay your needed procedure for one that is optional." Instead, her suggestion was to harvest my eggs between the first and second rounds of chemo.

I ignored the fact that she'd just described a fairly essential aspect of being a thirty-three-year-old woman as "optional," and stuck to the details. "I thought the rounds were once every twenty-one days, and I wouldn't even be able to start doing fertility until day six or so of that twenty-one-day countdown. Wouldn't that leave enough time?" This whole thing began to seem a little ridiculous. I'd been sick for so long without knowing it, and now suddenly I was on this insanely tight schedule. The calendar sitting in front of me began to feel like a prison sentence.

Dr. Levi was willing to extend to twenty-eight days. "But after that, if fertility is taking too long," she warned, "we would have to stop it and bring you back in for round two."

I tried another tack. "Aren't the steroids helping to contain the tumor right now? Couldn't I just stay on those until I'm done with fertility?"

She shook her head. "We're not going to agree to let you out of the hospital until you've gone through your first round of chemotherapy."

Finally, the bottom line.

I smashed my head against the little table filled with paperwork and confusion. I wasn't even sure I wanted children at all, but this entire conversation made me want to murder someone.

AS I GOT CLOSER to the MAKE A DECISION, DAMMIT deadline, panic took over. We were doing everything we could to make sure this was the best treatment possible, but we had no time to consider non-Western treatments or any other alternatives to the protocol as laid out by my medical team and verified by other Western doctors at cancer centers around the country.

I felt a complete lack of agency in the entire process. My health, my fertility, my body as I knew it—all were poised to be upended, and I could not do a single thing about it. My recipe for success had always included taking control of whatever was going on. Having no control over one of the most important decisions of my life left me utterly adrift. I had nothing familiar to grasp; I had no anchor. For the first time in my life, the best option in front of me was simply to submit to the circumstances engulfing me.

Enter my sister, with her years of hard-won experience fighting her own cancer. "I know it doesn't seem like you even have a choice, but you do," she said over the phone, understanding my attempt at explaining these unfamiliar feelings. "Either you can decide to surrender to their protocol and collaborate with them to make it work for you, or you can decide to be angry that you didn't have a choice and everything that's about to happen to you is someone else's fault." Then she told me she loved me very much. "You are my one and only sister. Please, for your sake, decide to own your treatment. Otherwise, you will spend the rest of your life, for however long you have, furious and miserable about 'those fucking doctors who ruined my life.'"

After sleeping on this conversation, I realized she was right. Surrendering to my treatment was the only way I could take ownership of my impossible situation.

ON FRIDAY, EIGHT DAYS after I was admitted to the hospital, I told my doctors we could start chemo on Sunday. I asked the onco-fertility specialist to set things up for whatever needed to happen with my ovaries on the following Friday. Elizabeth, her presence almost as constant as Michael's since our trip to the ER a week earlier, ran out to Michigan Avenue, found a bunch of GapBody items on sale, and came back with a sewing kit. We spent Saturday quietly altering the right sleeve of five different tops, so I could unsnap them and change my clothing without disconnecting my IV. We ate my favorite barbeque that night in an effort to celebrate my last day free of chemo.

Sunday started with a dose of Benadryl and my first medication—R, the antibody drug from my alphabet soup. Elizabeth and Michael watched me drift off to sleep as the IV slowly dripped its silent salvation. A few hours later when I woke up, the realization hit: I had just started a protocol that would do untold damage to my body in order to save it. Yet I had spent those first couple of hours calm enough to let the Benadryl put me to sleep. What my sister had said came back to me: By owning the decision, I had found the space to be calm. To be quiet. To surrender to the situation and the circumstances.

I took a bite of leftover beef brisket and dozed off again.

MICHAEL

MICHAEL CLAIMS WE first met when I was in eighth grade. I'm still not convinced. At that time in my life, boys—especially older, cute, popular, unattainable boys—were not yet on my radar. I attended an all-girls college preparatory school. Boys were out of sight, out of mind.

School was a world of cattiness and competition, with a solid dose of elitism mixed with self-esteem issues. In the hallowed halls of upper-crust Washington, DC, daily personal success was highly dependent upon a complex amalgam of natural ability, hard work, and political skill. Athleticism, beauty, wealth, brains, and personality all played roles too. I navigated my way through all this by using sarcasm as a wall, academic achievement as a goal, and soccer as a distraction. The fact that I loved math and wanted to build cool things, like skyscrapers and bridges and the next supercharged Ford Mustang, made me a bit of an oddity in this gilded microcosm.

We did have a "brother" school, located just on the other side of a huge field and a massive Episcopal church. (I still wonder at the intentionality of putting God between the sexes.) The boys at that school were a product of their own *Lord of the Flies*–type crucible. We would encounter them at scheduled rituals: seasonal school dances, rare joint church services, and infrequent coed classes—which were most certainly not scheduled until the girls' administration was positive that they would not interfere with our learning to talk for ourselves: eighth-grade drama, eleventh- and twelfth-grade English, math or science only with special permission.

My first memory of talking to Michael came near the end of tenth grade. I knew who he was—one of the smartest guys in his class, a go-to lead for school musicals, captain of the soccer team—but we had never really chatted. We did have a mutual friend, though: Benjamin. Both boys' parents worked in my school's administration, so both were fairly constant fixtures around my school. One day, as the entire girls' high school was coming out of an assembly on some women-empowerment topic, religious or otherwise, I noticed Benjamin and Michael leaning up against the wall, a wave of teenaged women crashing around them. One of the boys—I'm still not sure who—called my name.

I turned around.

Michael was waving a little white box in my direction. "I got you a present."

My priority just then was heading to lacrosse practice. But I walked up to them anyway, glanced at Benjamin (who shrugged and curved in on himself, distancing himself from the interaction without actually leaving), and accepted the gift. "Um, thanks. Not to be rude, because I always like presents, but . . . why did you get me one?"

His seventeen-year-old arrogance, born of brains, athletic ability, and a head of floppy blond hair, was already undermining the manners and modesty beaten into him by the diligence of a single mother, but he did have the grace to look a little sheepish.

"I saw it and thought of you. I just came back from snowboarding in Switzerland and thought you would enjoy it."

My eyebrows met my hairline. *WHAT? You're on a scholarship. How the hell did you just come back from snowboarding in Switzerland? Wait, you snowboard?* Suddenly, that made him super attractive to me. I had a vision of a snowboard-toting, black leather jacket–wearing blond stowing away on a plane to Switzerland. This was 1995, after all; only rebellious guys snowboarded back then. My reaction would have been similar if he'd told me that he rode a motorcycle and owned a pit bull.

I opened the box. Nestled inside, in a cocoon of white tissue paper, was a smaller plastic box holding a large piece of chocolate in the shape of an orange. I opened it up, turned the box over, and dropped the orange into my hand. It split open, into ten or twelve little sections. I'm not usually a giggler, but this little orange, so organized and endearing, made me giggle. I handed the box back to him and popped one of the sections into my mouth. It tasted like orangey, sugary, milky chocolate. I offered a section back to him, which he took, watching me carefully, and one to Benjamin, who declined, shrugged, and slouched off, his work as wingman clearly done. I closed the sections back in on themselves, making do without the two missing sections. Michael opened the box back up so I could drop the orange, still intact, back into its home. My hand brushed his as I took the box back from him. Clearly, it was a little gift from the airport in Switzerland, perhaps a total afterthought, but I was touched.

"Thank you." I looked up at him, noticing for the first time that his eyes were greenish-brown with flecks of yellow, not the blue I had been expecting.

"You're welcome. Can I walk you to lacrosse practice?"

That chocolate orange made us friends.

As our friendship evolved, Michael's group of friends became friends with my group of friends, and my group of friends started pairing off with his. Sometime that summer, I started dating one of the other boys in our group, a relationship that lasted until early fall. Ever the serial monogamist (as I would later learn), Michael remained curiously unattached the entire time. And we stayed friends.

Everything about our schools was designed to prepare students for the best colleges in the world, hopefully with a reasonably solid moral compass, a commitment to pursuing excellence, and a passion for something concrete, like music, arts, or athletics. Junior year was, predictably, brutal, consumed by college visits, SATs, AP examinations, desperate attempts to elevate GPAs as high as possible, and securing a final milestone in a sports championship or musical endeavor. The first semester of senior year was hardly different, with the added bonus of actually applying to colleges.

This is the moment where we all found ourselves. The boys in our group were seniors and sprinting down the homestretch. The girls were juniors and just beginning the slog. Needless to say, we were all a little stressed. Except for Michael. He was the only one who appeared untouched by the chaos.

This was in stark contrast to my own way of handling the stress, which involved a weekly *Holy shit, how am I going to get all of this done and done perfectly?* panic attack. I've always been grateful that my school did not give out A+ grades, because if I had gotten "only" an A instead of an A+, there would have been a catastrophic internal meltdown.

Michael was being aggressively recruited by an inordinate number of top colleges and always seemed entirely at ease, whereas if I didn't get early admission into Brown University, my life was OVER.

I was a horse with blinders. From the very start, my love for Brown was a little irrational, born of the first sight of intense green grass against the bright brick. My entire career at my prep school, starting in kindergarten, was geared toward getting me into one of the best colleges in the world. I had no other ideas, partially because I'd never been told by either my parents or my school that I could have any other ideas. *You can do whatever you want with your life* was always couched in *after you go to college*. Riding along on this tide of someone else's creation, I pushed my brain and my body to achieve what was needed, and periodically released some of the tension through a yellow card on the soccer field or a private anxiety attack.

By junior year, I was feeling the crushing pressure of it all. Michael's calmness drew me closer. We started talking on the phone more frequently and asking little favors of each other. We would find ourselves separating from the others whenever we were out.

And then one day, Michael asked me to pick him up from the airport. He was heading out for a few days to the University of Chicago for a recruiting visit and needed a ride home. Or so he claimed. Never mind that he had his own car and a doting mother. He asked, and I was game.

On the way back to his house that Sunday evening in late September, we stopped at a Pizzeria Uno that no longer exists in downtown Bethesda. We ordered, and Michael disappeared to the bathroom. On the table, he had left his notepad. Michael always had a notepad with him and a Bic blue ballpoint pen tucked behind his ear. Despite the fact that constantly writing down thoughts and ideas is akin to social suicide in high school, he could get away with it because he easily moved between all of the cliques—popular, athletic, musical, artistic, nerdy. I never really thought about it one way or the other, it was simply part of who he was.

After a moment or so of looking around the room and sucking up Coke through my straw, I picked up his notepad and started flipping through it. Knowing that this was a gross invasion of his privacy didn't stop me, but only made me glance up more frequently to see if he was coming back. As expected, it was mostly just a bunch of notes: thoughts about the University of Chicago, his itinerary, some early drafts of various college essays, a few lists of schools and soccer coaches and other contacts . . . and a draft letter to me.

What?

I immediately stopped paying attention to the bathroom door and started reading in earnest. I know I have a copy of this note somewhere in my box of memories, but I much prefer my recollection of it, which is infused with the intensity and emotion I felt upon discovering this unlikely document.

> Dear Lydia . . . friendship has grown into something more . . . not sure what to say because I don't want to ruin what we have . . . Your relationship over the summer made it more obvious to me that you're more than a friend . . . You think I have it all figured out, but I don't . . . I never tell anyone this, but I want to tell you . . . don't know . . . but . . .

Pain. In the note, I read intense pain. There was the pain from unrequited desire, but it was more than that. Suddenly, he was more than just a rock for me to lean against. He was a rock with cracks and faults. All the while I had been depending on him for his steadiness, he'd been leaning on me to calm his own inner agony. I realized then that Michael needed a part of me I didn't even know I had.

And then Michael was standing next to the table, with a look on his face that vacillated between storming out of the restaurant and sitting down to see how this disaster would play out. He sat down.

I flipped his notepad back to the top page and slid it across the table. "Sorry," I mumbled sheepishly. "None of that was any of my business."

He flipped back to the *Dear Lydia* letter and sighed. "Well, now you know. What do you want to do about it?"

The pizza showed up, and we both took the opportunity to gather ourselves while pulling slices of hot, gooey deliciousness onto our plates. I started eating mine and contemplated his question. His stayed on his plate.

"Is your friend who I dated over the summer going to flip

out?" First things first: logistics before feelings. *Anything* before feelings.

"I'll deal with that, but probably not." His slice remained whole.

I liberated another slice from the pie. "Will this ruin our friendship?"

"Probably. But honestly, I've gotten to the point where I don't think I can be friends with you anymore either way."

"What? Why?" Alarm flashed through my chest unlike anything I had ever felt. I'd come to rely on him so completely that the thought of not being friends with him lanced my heart. I had no way to cope with this revelation other than to set aside my pizza and stare at him.

"Lydia, for as smart as you are, you can be remarkably stupid," he grumbled. "I've come to rely on you too, you know."

"For what you wrote about in your letter?" I asked, pointing to the pad of paper. "But I don't understand. You're always so"—I scrambled for the right word—"whole. I feel like I'm the needy one. I've never quite understood why you were friends with me in the first place. There's nothing you need from me." I spread my arms out to show him that they were empty.

"You have no idea who you are, do you?"

I stared at him, appalled. Of course I knew who I was. I was insecure, a control freak. I was athletic and smart. I was sarcastic and could be cruel. I didn't need anything. Except . . .

A scene from earlier that month blazed in my mind. I had a paper due, a book to read, a lab to complete, and my brain had locked. I couldn't start my to-do list because I was overwhelmed by my to-do list. Michael had found me weeping quietly at a table in the library, surrounded by papers. He had laughed, given me a hug, and helped me prioritize. Then he sat with me, doing his own homework while I did mine, chuckling every now and again despite my fierce, recurring glare.

Apparently, this guy sitting across from me had snuck under my armor when I wasn't looking and started to soothe my frayed edges.

"You're beautiful and kind," he began. "You would lay down in traffic for any of your friends. You are incredibly strong and forceful, and you don't let anyone treat you or anyone you love poorly." He grinned. "Sure, it sometimes makes you a bitch, but it's amazing to watch." Then he paused, sobering. "Your strength is soothing to me. Half the time, I don't know what I'm doing, and it scares the shit out of me. But then I look over at you and something . . . just . . . shifts."

"Um . . ." And then I burst out laughing. My only thought was that it was better than crying. I had no idea what to do with such honesty. "So we can't be friends anymore." It wasn't really a question.

"Nope. I mean, seriously, if you find dating me that awful, I could figure out how to maybe downshift how I feel about you. But why not give this a shot?"

Why not, indeed?

"Right, dating you would be terrible," I replied. "I mean, you're hot and athletic and super smart and sweet, and I already spend most of my time with you anyway."

He grinned and started eating his pizza, knowing that victory was in sight.

"But what do I do when we fall apart? Because we will, you know. You'll find someone else, and then where the hell will I be?"

"No, I won't." It was so simple and, at that moment, so obvious—and looking back on it, such a wonderful thing for a seventeen-year-old to say. "I'm not going to find anyone else who makes me feel the way you do."

I looked at him, and he looked at me, and I felt the quicksand of young love take hold.

FROM THAT EVENING forward, we were *that* couple. The amount of time we spent together went from *most* to *always*, and we were unabashed about how it delighted both of us. It was so intense that the senior girls that year put a picture of us from some school dance in the yearbook with a thick, black *X* through it.

Michael applied early to Brown, in part because he knew that's where I wanted to go. And with his résumé and charisma, he got in. He then made sure that I kept my grades up so I could join him a year later. Our conversations remained as honest and revealing as they were that first night over pizza. And I loved every minute of it. The intensity, the dramatic mood swings, the craziness of being desperately, deeply in love for the first time—it blew me away.

This intoxicating joy lasted until a few weeks before he left for college. Then, for reasons he couldn't verbalize and I couldn't define, he shifted. His carefully constructed exterior began to show cracks: A fight in his basement about how I should just leave him because he was a fraud. A moment at a friend's house when he showed up late, terrified about being left out of whatever juvenile silliness was happening. Brief moments of tenderness were intertwined with increasingly baffling behavior.

Michael left for Brown in August. For the first few weeks, we chatted on the phone about school and soccer, and I started learning about college life. My sister, who had taken a year off after high school, was also a freshman, so between the two of them, I was taking a secondhand crash course in college. And frankly, I didn't much like what I was witnessing. Classes aside, both Corinna and Michael were snowed under, confused, and trying desperately to find their footing.

Michael started pulling away. Our calls became shorter and less frequent. More and more often, when I called, he would be unavailable. When he did call, it was always with an air of distraction.

I saw him once that autumn, when I visited Princeton for the Brown–Princeton soccer game. He was frayed. Physically, he looked exhausted and a little wild-eyed; spiritually and emotionally, he seemed to be gasping for air. He tumbled into my arms like he was escaping from jail and spent much of our brief afternoon together sleeping with his head in my lap while I stared at a tree, bewildered and heartsick. He lost his temper badly during the soccer game, something I'd never seen him do. Afterward, he went north on I-95 to Rhode Island while I turned south toward DC.

Thanksgiving wasn't much better. Michael came home with a goatee and a healthy appetite for alcohol, both of which made him almost foreign to me. My dad tried to ease my concern by sharing some of his outrageous drinking stories from college, underscoring the message that it was all normal.

I kept working as hard as ever at school and sent in my early application to Brown. Maybe if I got in, we would be us again. One evening, a phone call blew out that candle.

"Slaby's just down the hall," his roommate claimed, but it was five minutes before Michael came to the phone, which seemed odd.

"Hi! How goes it?" I said.

"Oh, fine," Michael replied. "But I have a ton of work to do, and someone is having a party later. Can we chat tomorrow?"

A version of this conversation had been happening most times we got on the phone, and I was tired of it.

"No, we can't talk tomorrow, because we won't talk tomorrow," I snapped. "What the hell is going on with you? You're never around when I call, and when you are, you get off the phone as quickly as you can. You had a chance to break up with me when you were home for Thanksgiving. If this is what we are now, why didn't you just do it then?"

My stomach was in knots. The last thing I wanted was to lose him, but he was already gone. I didn't have anything to lose by pushing him.

"I loved the time we had together over Thanksgiving." His voice was low. I could practically hear his brain trying to figure out a response to my frustration.

"So why are you disappearing now? You're only there for another couple of weeks before winter break."

Nothing. I could hear him breathing, so I knew he was there.

"Mike? What's going on? Why won't you talk to me?"

I heard someone calling his name.

"I really have to go." He was distracted, talking quickly.

"No, you don't. If you get off the phone right now without telling me what's going on with you, don't bother calling me when you get home for Christmas."

I heard his name again. Closer. Louder. A girl's voice. Insisting.

He covered the phone, muffling his response. A door slammed, and the background noise dropped.

I sat quietly on my bed, waiting for him to return to the phone, to me.

"Things have changed," he said.

I stayed quiet.

"I've started spending a lot of time with a girl down the hall, and it's turning into something more."

I locked down. "Turning? Or turned? If you're in the middle of telling me that you're cheating on me with some cheap blonde, then you better be real specific about it." He was so far away, and I was just a teenager, broken-hearted and angry. My voice came out like a sharp slap, and I felt him recoil.

"Fine. We've been sleeping together since before Thanksgiving. Happy?"

"I can't believe you didn't have the courage to tell me the truth in person. I can't believe you've been letting me worry about you during this whole thing. I can't believe who you've turned into. Go. Fuck. Yourself."

I hung up, crawled under my covers, and stayed there for the rest of the winter.

MY SOCCER SEASON ended with a championship that I barely registered.

And then, shortly before Christmas, came a thin envelope with the Brown University seal in the upper-left corner. I sat in the front garden, having received it straight from the mailman, and opened it.

Congratulations, I am delighted . . .

How could I go there now that he was there? I decided to think about it after a nap.

In the days that followed, my friends and I symbolically burned all of our college application paperwork and stopped paying attention at school. I heard whispered conversations about how I was fading away from friendships. I only laughed when I was with my friends—and at the wrong moments. Some of them pointed out that I'd lost weight, which I hadn't even noticed, although it was obvious when I regarded myself carefully in the mirror.

A few of us convinced our parents to let us take a couple of "sick days" to go to Mardi Gras in New Orleans. We were met by friends at the airport with a handle of vodka, and my memories of what follows are disjointed. I was stuffed full of chocolate cake and gumbo. Bars accepted our 18-year-old IDs, granting us access to shots and cute boys who weren't going to be around long enough to break any hearts.

When I returned home, I showed up at lacrosse practice to find out my coach had replaced me as starting defensive wing. I was a senior, and a sophomore had taken my place on the field. I lost my temper and quit the team. I would go home at 3:30 p.m. and sleep until dinner, barely eat, do the minimum amount of homework so I wouldn't fail, and return to bed. On the weekends, I would often arise for the first time at nearly 4 p.m. when a friend would call to discuss plans for the evening.

I kept losing weight.

A doctor told me I had contracted mono. A therapist told me I had mild depression. All I knew was I wanted to sleep all the time, curled up with my cat, and I didn't care why.

As winter yielded to spring, I regained resilience. I resolved to be delighted that I was going to Brown, that all of my hard work had paid off to send me to the school that had entranced me from the moment I first stepped onto its Main Green, when I had looked at my mother, driving me on the obligatory junior-year tour of beautiful campuses of higher education, and said, "This is it." My mother had stayed quiet, as she always did, careful not to inject her own thoughts into my deeply personal decision. I had felt a kinetic connection to Brown. The idea of it both nurtured and challenged my budding sense of self and purpose.

In this fit of determination, I attended the annual A Day on College Hill—a preorientation program for admitted students. I tried hard not to conjure a run-in with Michael, but there was no way we wouldn't reconnect. Despite the anger and hurt, Michael and I were two magnets, each tuned to the other. As I walked across the Main Green, I saw him sitting on a staircase eating his lunch. We locked eyes.

We agreed to have a chat. As we sat in a park near campus, looking out over the sunset—and perhaps channeling some of the sun's eternal metaphor about possibility and renewal—Michael tried to apologize but couldn't find the words. He, too, had lost weight, and he looked even more frayed and wild-eyed than he had in the fall. His nature, always centered and self-assured, had fundamentally shifted. His confidence in his athletic and academic abilities was diminished. The faults and cracks I had noticed that night over pizza, a million years ago, had taken over his entire nature.

I was helpless.

My heart broke anew. This man who was not perfect, but who was in so many ways perfect for me, had shifted down a path that made little sense to either of us, and scared the shit out of both of us. He knew it. I knew it. And our collective fear connected us that night. As we identified this fear in each other, we fell back into our own easy comfort, which brought each of us a measure of calm. We walked back to campus hand in hand, and our intense relief at the reconnection was captured in photos that disappeared shortly after they materialized. When we met up with some of his friends, they hugged me with abandon and whispered into my ear, "Thank God you're here. Please help him."

Our tender reconciliation was short-lived. The day after I left, he returned to the girl down the hall.

Michael came home from college to a summer job, and I left to work with dolphins in Hawaii, sleeping on my cousin's floor. When I returned, Michael and I had our worst fight yet. The lingering angst of a yearlong breakup finally overcame me, and I snapped. Who knows what we actually said to each other, but the explosion left emotions, accusations, and pieces of our broken hearts littered throughout his mother's basement. I drove home in tears, taking an hour to drive what usually took twenty minutes.

At 8:00 a.m. the following morning, my mom handed me the phone. It was Michael's mother, begging me to come to the hospital. After I'd left the night before, Michael had wrapped his car around a tree while trying to follow me home. He was refusing to see anyone until he saw me. So I waded back into the quagmire, worried and battling my own frustration and sadness in the face of his crisis.

In his hospital room, his broken right leg was a woeful presence on the bed, and his right arm was in a cast. His IV stand was filled with empty bags of saline and full bags of pain medications. Stunned at this real-life version of a scene from *ER*, I carefully navigated tubes and casts and machinery to sit beside him. As I looked at my person, the reality of Medical Crisis drove away all the Very Important Reasons to hate him.

His mother fretted and hovered at the door. A nurse bustled in to swap out an empty saline bag and said, echoing the comments of his college friends, "Thank God you're here. He's been an absolute nightmare waiting for you."

I waited for her to leave before leaning over him. "Did you do this to make me come back?"

Michael grimaced, neither affirming nor denying.

I stood up and walked out as his mother, no longer able to contain herself, broke through the invisible barrier at the door and flew to her only child's side. I stumbled into the hallway's nearest chair and held my head in my hands until Michael's best friend showed up, remarking, "I'm surprised it took this long for us all to be meeting around Mike's hospital bed."

His clear-eyed honesty hit me like a punch in the gut.

The next day, I came back with reinforcements. My mother stood by the door as I sat down on Michael's bed and took his hand—the one without the cast.

"Christ, child, you look like shit." Mom has never been one to mince words.

Michael had the good humor to smile.

"I'll leave you two. Five minutes, Lydia."

"Thanks, Mom," I called after her, grateful for her stability and support.

He looked up at me. "You're leaving, aren't you?" His voice was quiet, laced with pain and dulled by drugs.

I stared at the face of the boy-turning-man whom I loved so indelibly that I could barely breathe. "We can't keep doing this . . . this . . . dance of pain and love, and staying and going. It's going to end up killing one of us. It very nearly killed you. And I couldn't ever live with that."

"I don't want to live without you." He stated it as a fact. No agenda, just the fact.

"Well, you need to figure it out. Between your lying and cheating and turning into someone I don't recognize, you've made it impossible for us to be together. And this crap"—I waved around the hospital room—"of using my love for you to pull me back in, ends now. You made the choice to leave me, now you have to learn to live with it."

Before he could say anything, I kissed him hard on the lips, gently on his hand, and walked out the door. He still says it's the bravest thing he's ever seen anyone do.

GRACE

THE IDEA OF GRACE, a Christian theory, is one I've never fully understood. Combine it with aspects of Eastern thought, though, and it becomes a lovely moment of utter stillness and calm achieved through full acceptance of reality as it currently exists. I am not a theologian and have no desire to be, but in my experience, pain—whether it's physical, mental, or emotional—becomes more bearable when I accept that pain for what it is and stay present inside it.

Dr. Levi had warned me that the time between rounds one and two of my chemotherapy protocol was going to be, in some ways, the worst of the entire four months. Side effects build up, so even though hair loss and exhaustion would be at their most potent by the end of the entire protocol, the shock of experiencing the various consequences for the first time would be worse. We had just flooded my body with dozens of new chemicals and medications, and if I was going to react to any of them negatively, it would happen after round one.

Promises, promises.

Two days after I got home from my two-week hospital sentence and stopped taking the prednisone, my body exploded into hives. It took another two days to determine the cause: an "essential" prescription designed to help my kidneys process the dying cancer cells. It rapidly became "nonessential," and we controlled the reaction. By that point, I was so excited to be neither in the hospital nor at the whim of my itchy skin that I actually did a bunch of work and laid out a plan with a colleague for a small project I wanted to complete a few days later. At the time, I felt compelled and delighted to feel productive and useful. I needed something bigger than my itchy skin and incomprehensible tumor to remind me of the vast world that existed beyond the confines of my body. I went to bed that night thrilled that I had beaten the odds with a bad, but easily solvable, reaction to one of my medications.

I should have knocked on wood. Or clonked my head against a door.

At 5:15 the following morning I was already awake, still not recovered from the jet lag of leaving the hospital's time zone, when a pain unlike anything I've ever experienced started emanating from inside my hips. In a panic, I texted Corinna to find out what the hell was going on.

"You're having bony pain," she texted back. "Call me."

It turns out that a drug I'd been given, Neulasta, helps stimulate red and white blood cell production in order to rebuild white blood cell counts. It (or something similar) was "necessary" in order to ensure that my immune system would not be completely wiped out and to allow treatment to continue on a reasonably predictable schedule. Neulasta is time-released over seven days (the daily version is called Neupogen), and at 5:15 a.m., it had officially activated.

What was occurring was dramatic bone marrow stimulation, which causes the bone marrow to expand inside my bones where there is no room for it to expand given the lack of elasticity and flexibility within those sturdy pieces that hold our bodies upright. Hence the term *bony pain*. This is such a well-known side effect of the process that it has a name. That, Dr. Levi (for very good reasons) didn't warn me about.

Corinna explained all this to me, sharing that absolutely nothing can be done for the pain except distract myself by watching *Super Troopers*. Weeping, I got off the phone and did a sweep of the apartment for anything that could dull the pain.

I immediately went through all options in both the medicine and the liquor cabinets: full bottle of Aleve . . . expired oxycodone from someone's dental history . . . bottles of Johnnie Walker, Glenfiddich, and red wine. The thought of getting drunk was tempting, but after contemplating it for about five minutes, I decided that would be worse than the pain. So instead I paced.

And paced.

And paced.

Two Aleve, an oxycodone, and two hours later, I was on my way to Dr. Levi, hobbling and shuffling as I leaned against Michael, gritting my teeth and still weeping, and pissed at how woozy I was from the oxycodone. The look of pity on my doorman's face is still seared into my brain.

Dr. Levi took one look at me and put me in an exam room to hide my pain from the patients in the communal infusion room. She set up an IV drip of steroids and fluids, intended to diminish the inflammatory response that continued to pulse through the large bones of my hips, sacrum, and upper thighs, and now had also migrated into my shoulders. The doctor wrote out a new prescription for oxycodone and told me to sit tight and wait for the pain to pass.

I don't remember much of that day. I remember Michael disappearing to fill the prescription, then coming back with salvation in an orange plastic bottle. I remember fading in and out of consciousness when the pain got bad enough that my mind simply shut down. I vividly recall the crunch of the paper on the medical exam table as I shifted. I was most comfortable lying in a fetal position, curled up on my right side. Every now and again, I would stretch out my legs. My arms were wrapped around my stomach as if, without them, my guts would just ooze out of my body and spill, warm and steaming, onto the floor. Michael, for the most part, either stood or sat beside me, holding my right hand as it clenched my left ribs. He would occasionally look at his email on his phone, but otherwise he just sat.

Halfway through this dreadful day, I got my period. Usually, such an ill-timed gift would have pushed me into object-throwing hysterics, but the pain combined with the powerful, opiate-induced haziness resulted simply in more tears. They streamed down my face, pooling with my snot in my ears and hair. I shuffled out to the bathroom, asking all the nurses on the way if anyone had a pad—I couldn't handle the thought of a tampon. One did. It took all of my focus to unwrap the pad, peel away its backing, press it into my underwear, securely wrap the wings around the cotton, and pull everything back into place. I wondered if this was the last period I would ever get and had a small moment of clarity where I could chuckle at the absurdity of such a milestone.

As the day wore on and the drugs did nothing to lessen the pain, I realized when I stayed conscious and fully focused on the present moment filled with pain, it lessened on its own. The minute I started thinking outside of my immediate experience and surroundings, the pain would flare up again, threatening to pull me back into physical and mental agony. To stay sane, I had to fully accept the reality of where I was and simply submit to it. Grace.

When the hospital shows you that preposterous *How bad is your pain level?* diagram, with the happy face over the 1 and the face in absolute agony over the 10, I was, for the first time in my life, solidly registering a 10. Staying present with the pain would lessen it to perhaps 9.5, but that 0.5 was enough to give me the space to breathe a little deeper or unclench my shoulders just a tiny bit. In that space, I could sit inside the pain without needing to crawl out the window and free fall twenty-one stories to the sidewalk below. Finding that tiny moment of grace took me outside of the pain and let me focus on my breath as it moved in and out of my nose. On my husband's face, beautiful and etched with concern. On the feeling of my hand moving, fingers bending. On the touch of his hand, like soft, uncompromising love and devotion. On the wall of the room, pure white and almost glowing. On a bird swooping outside the window, reveling in the joy of moving through the air. Staying present at a 9.5 pain level felt like a gift from above.

By 3 p.m., Dr. Levi was forced to reassess. No matter how much grace I was able to harness, my pain was not going anywhere. The doctor decided to admit me to the hospital, where I could receive IV drugs. While making the call and typing in the order, she explained that this level of pain happens about 5 percent of the time with the time-released version of the drug, so next time we would switch to the daily version. In the meantime, we simply had to wait out the next few days while the drug ran its course. I could barely comprehend her words.

I shuffled into a wheelchair, and Michael wheeled me out of her office, into the elevator, down nineteen floors, across the sky bridge, and into the admissions area of the main hospital. We waited. Not the first time that day, staying present was a fleeting wish. I started to freak out, fully convinced that I would never reach the final step: sweet oblivion.

With the fruitless opiates churning in my stomach, I looked at Michael, who looked at the admissions staff, and I was wheeled to my favorite nurse, Stacy, and my favorite tech, Theo, in my favorite cancer ward, just before I puked all over the place.

In short order, I was injected with stronger opiates and a heavy-duty anti-inflammatory. The relief was instant, an all-engulfing void left by the complete absence of pain. Time stood still. I had moved from the wheelchair to the edge of the bed in order to receive the injections just a few minutes earlier—except that Michael clocked it at just under an hour. Stacy took my blood pressure and asked me various questions, which I answered quietly, but I don't remember a minute of it. I just remember the agony and then, like a flood, the relief. Now I'm able to grasp how people can sit and meditate for hours. It probably doesn't feel like hours; it just feels like quiet bliss.

That evening, Michael convinced Stacy to look the other way

while he moved my fertility medicine into the patient refrigerator and injected me with hormones. Theo fussed over me, snugly tucking in my sheets and taking my blood pressure more than was strictly necessary. Elizabeth magically appeared. I kept my dinner down.

Later that night, I ran my hand through my hair and came away with a clump of eighteen-inch hairs lying in my hand like weird skinny snakes. I no longer had the energy or self-control to keep my brain calm, and I let my worst fear overpower me: Michael would take a good, hard look at his sick, drugged, infertile, emaciated, balding wife and decide this was absolutely not worth it. He would just walk out of the hospital and my life forever.

Hysterics completely demolished me. Michael tried holding me. He tried talking to me. I had no strength to push him away, but my mind wouldn't let his presence convince me. Finally, he played the song "Ho Hey" by The Lumineers on repeat, and the singers' rhythmic chorus began to pacify me, filtering through my drugged mind:

> I belong with you, you belong with me,
> you're my sweetheart . . .
>
> I belong with you, you belong with me,
> you're my sweet . . .

I drifted off to sleep.

Later that night, I bolted upright in bed, panic swarming yet again, but this time with no focus. It was simple adrenaline, coursing through my system. I couldn't tamp it down or stay still inside it. I was sore, but it was under control. I didn't want to wake up Michael. So I quietly got out of bed, grabbed my computer, and went down the hall to the lounge where I could work on something for the office.

A few hours later, Stacy found me, waving the next injections like a New Yorker chasing down a cab in rush hour. "WHAT ARE YOU DOING?" she shouted.

I burst into tears and tried to explain my fight-or-flight reaction. "I have no idea where it came from or why it's still here. I can't sleep. My hair is falling out. I need to do this thing for the office, but I can barely focus on it. This whole thing is . . . insane!"

She sat down next to me, removed my computer from my lap, saved and closed the document on the screen, and set it down. Then she gave me my medication and sat back against the couch, watching me.

"Here's the deal. Some people have an adverse reaction to opiates," she explained. "This means that after you've been on them for some amount of time, instead of calming you down, they spin you up. You're still woozy, but instead of wanting to sleep, you want to crawl up the walls." Apparently this is a known side effect of the drug. But Stacy felt I was taking a minor adverse reaction and exacerbating it considerably. "Why are you working at four in the morning when you are clearly woozy from opiates?"

"I need to get this stuff done," I answered, "and nothing else was calming me down."

"And are you calmer now?"

Touché. "No, because I wasn't doing a very good job at it.

Because I'm super woozy." Tears of frustration trickled down my face.

"Do you actually need to get it done?"

My smile disrupted the flood. "No. My colleague said that he would do the whole thing in the morning, and I should throw my computer out the window. But I wanted to help! I feel so useless right now."

"There is absolutely nothing useless about taking the time you need to heal." She took my hand in hers. "I hate to break this to you, but you have cancer."

I glared at her, moving my hand back to my thigh. "You think I don't know that?"

She looked at me with kindness in her eyes. "I wonder if you really do, seriously. Your body is fighting a tumor the size of a grapefruit. Your heart is working really hard to beat, even though this tumor is practically sitting on it. Your various systems are handling at least a dozen exceedingly powerful drugs. On top of all of this, you're taking fertility medications. And now you're spending brain power and energy on everything and everyone in your life except for you."

She confessed that she'd overheard some of my conversation with Michael. "I can't believe that you think he would leave you in the middle of all this. Do you have any idea how he looks at you? Do you know how many husbands *don't* spend the night here with their wives? What you guys have is something I rarely see. The other nurses and doctors have been commenting on it. Seriously, you just need to calm down."

Could I? Sure, I had learned how to meditate before I came into the hospital. But could I really calm down? Could I do what my body and my mind needed—every day, day in and day out? Although I didn't want to admit it, the answer was quite obviously no.

Meditation isn't sleep. I was sleeping a lot, not meditating. I was escaping, not actively calming my mind and body. Sure, I had moments where I was able to meditate, but it seemed like such a weak counterforce to the perpetual despair, panic, and fear—for my life, my marriage, my sense of self. I often lost the train of quiet as the panic whelmed once more.

I inhaled a big breath. She rubbed my back. I breathed again. And again. My eyelids fluttered. Stacy picked up my computer, offered me her hand, and put me back to bed. Where I slept.

DESPITE OUR BEST EFFORTS, including sneaking drugs into the hospital and continuing to search for fat deposits to use as injection sites on my rapidly shrinking body, fertility treatments didn't work. According to a voicemail left by the least empathetic nurse I had yet to encounter, various numbers weren't breaking all the right thresholds, so I was told to stop the injections and call with any questions. It was akin to a break-up by Post-it note.

I picked up this message while receiving fluids in Dr. Levi's office, so of course I rapidly flagged her down to accuse her of ripping my fertility out of my body like a priest at an exorcism.

"You've only had one round of treatment," she countered. "I *promise* that your ovaries are doing just fine. But in the past three weeks, you've had chemotherapy drugs, antibiotics, antifungals, antivirals, steroids, Neulasta and the debacle and drugs associated with dealing with that . . ." The list went on: An allergic reaction and the medications and madness. Fertility drugs and an allergic reaction to one of those. The stress of having my life turned upside-down. And, as icing on the cake, I was probably now under 5 percent body fat. "My guess is that your body, quite intelligently, has prioritized which drugs it will pay attention to and which drugs to just pass through," Dr. Levi continued. "I'm not surprised that the fertility medications didn't make the cut. Let's give you the shot to shut everything down and then wait it out. You'll be fine. I promise."

That was the phrase I focused on: *You'll be fine. I promise.*

HAIR OPTIONAL

ABOUT A YEAR BEFORE cancer came into my life, Michael and I adopted Ellie and Jake from a working farm in Michigan. We were told they were eight weeks old, but our new veterinarian set us straight. Ellie, at thirteen ounces, was the runt of the five-week-old collection, so small that she could comfortably fit in the palm of my hand. Jake suffered from "wobbly cat syndrome," an underdeveloped cerebellum caused by in-utero exposure to distemper.

We brought them home, and I built them a house out of an old cardboard wardrobe box. Then I spent the next eight weeks studying for the Illinois bar exam, three feet from them at all times. From the moment we brought them into the car, they became an integral part of our lives. We taught them to eat, using droppers and pureed chicken and endless patience. They visited the vet six times in the first week as we learned how to keep them alive. I didn't sleep for two days and didn't eat for four as I cradled these tiny lives in my hands and heart. I watched Michael fall in love with what he called the "furry midgets." I called them "the babies."

When I came home from the hospital after two weeks in chemo, bruised and exhausted (and smelling like a pharmacy, I'm sure), the babies had just celebrated their first birthday. Jake wobbled less; Ellie was still only the size of a large kitten. As I toppled into bed that first night back, beyond grateful to be in my own bed with my husband, Jake curled up at my feet and Ellie by my head, and that's how we stayed for the entirety of my treatment.

From them, I learned how to rest. They would stay in bed with me, not eating, on the days when I couldn't find the strength to do anything else but my brain was telling me otherwise. I would sit up, intending to satiate my brain's need to be productive, and one or both of them would roll over, swat me, and go back to sleep, persuading me to do the same.

On the days when I did have the energy to move about, the babies would wake up in the morning and get off the bed, walking over me or prodding me as they went. If I still hadn't moved after a few moments, Ellie would come back and yowl at me until I got up. We would spend half an hour on something, and then the three of us would curl up on the couch for a midmorning nap, the babies curled up between my knees, having learned that my hot flashes were unpredictable.

Ellie and Jake are still my greatest teachers as I learn to listen to my own body. I would watch them watching me, and after a few months, I began to see the little cues that they recognized from the very beginning. Lethargy versus true exhaustion. Busy brain versus quiet body. They also taught me how to nap. I learned the importance of being able to nap whenever needed, even if circumstances would seem to discourage it. To this day, when I need a day of rest, Michael still compares me to a cat.

DURING THOSE FIRST few weeks in the hospital, I would smash out thousand-word emails to my family and friends, giving them the most recent details of my diagnosis and treatment and casually mentioning my love of dark chocolate. One day at home, as I pounded away at the screen of my iPad, Michael asked what I was working on.

When I told him, he replied, "How many emails have you sent?"

"I dunno . . . maybe six or seven?" I shrugged and kept typing. (It took me a few years to learn that my thoughts tended to be the length of book chapters.)

"Maybe it's time we did something useful with your compulsive need to be writing about all this." Michael, with his superpower for all things tech and digital design, had channeled his own distress about my health into website development. He'd created three websites already, and I could tell from the gobbledygook on his screen that he was working on a fourth.

"I *am* doing something useful with my compulsive need to be writing about all this. I'm writing about all this."

"You're also hijacking people's inboxes." As the recipient of hundreds of emails a day, Michael thinks about these things, which is very kind of him. At that particular moment, though, I found it exceedingly irritating.

"Seriously? They don't have to read my email if they don't want to. It's not like their inbox is holding a gun to their head. What the fuck, man? Will you just let me write to my people?"

He held his hands up in protest. "Sorry! I didn't mean it that way. I just meant, if you have so much to say about all this, maybe you should just start a blog. I could help you create it. And that would give people a break from your emails."

I glared at him. "Have you heard from people? Are they annoyed?"

"'Annoyed' is the wrong word. You're very . . . descriptive. It can be overwhelming." He studiously avoided looking at me.

A blog. Huh. A blog implies *public*. I wasn't sure I was a fan of that.

"You do know that people are already forwarding your emails to friends and colleagues, so it's not like those are private."

"They're doing *what*?" I was appalled—and yet a little proud of myself. Fame is very conflicting.

He ignored me. "I've bought you a bunch of addresses. We already have lydiaslaby.com, but you might want to call the blog something different. And you should use Wordpress—there are some good templates that you might like."

I began to wonder exactly who this blog was for.

But then I realized it was a project we could do together, something positive and dynamic and creative in this land of depressing hospital and destructive medicine, of waiting to get better . . . or worse. And besides, if people were already sharing my emails, what difference did it really make?

"Is hairoptional.com available?" I asked. Lately, I'd discovered I was secretly delighted with my bald head. Still, I didn't want this to be something just for cancer people.

He clicked and typed and scanned. "Yup."

MUCH TO MY simultaneous delight and aggravation, Michael was right about the blog.

As the influx of information slowed and we found ourselves

in the new normal of cancer treatment, my brain felt less overwhelmed. Michael—realizing the crisis was, in a sense, over—went back to his day job of getting a president elected for the second time. As a result, I took over the note-taking about my illness and treatment. I also began processing (in therapy and on my computer screen) what was happening to me and my life.

The blog was entirely for me. I didn't write it for an audience beyond people who care about me. Weirdly enough, though, more than just my people seemed to really like it. Go figure.

One particularly frustrating day, I titled a post:

GO HOME. STAY THERE. OPEN WINDOW.

Every year I promise myself that our next home will have windows that actually, truly open. Windows like I had in my office at the Massachusetts Statehouse where on particularly beautiful mornings, I would climb up on my windowsill and pull the window up six or seven feet (and it still wouldn't be fully open) and just stand there, inside yet outside, letting the cool, soft, morning air wash over me. Just stand there, hearing the traffic from Beacon and Park, smelling the wind that had just ruffled the trees in the Common, simply feeling the morning in my small corner of Boston.

The smaller version that I grew up with in a historic row house would work too. But windows, with panes, that actually let air into the building, have been something that I've been promising myself for a while. Instead, I'm on the forty-eighth floor of a high rise with views that stretch to both Iowa and Wisconsin, with windows that don't ventilate. Trade-offs.

So my doctor's instructions this morning, written on my lab results, in all caps: "GO HOME. STAY THERE. OPEN WINDOW." smarted a bit, especially because Chicago is having one of those summer days that compel you to be outside. If it were January, the temperature would be -30 degrees and kids would be kept home to prevent death by freezing cold wind. But it's August, so we have a beautiful, 70 degree breeze with white caps on the lake and tourists wandering around confused, because they thought they were in Chicago, not San Diego.

I'm neutropenic, which basically means that my white blood count has gone well below normal (normal range: 4.5–10. I'm at 0.15). This is normal for post chemo; it's just the last time I had these counts, I was in the hospital, delirious with bony pain and various opiates, so I didn't pay much attention to it. The drugs that give me bony pain are designed to prevent the numbers from going that low, or at least help them recover faster if they do. The dull, aching throb in my pelvis and femurs for the last few days tells me that the medicine is doing something, but apparently not enough.

Because I'm me, I'm cheating and writing this while sitting on my balcony (too windy to read out here), but I'm on lockdown for a couple days.

Other than that, things have been going well. I was released from the hospital Sunday, went to see Of Monsters and Men and Florence and the Machine

> at Lollapalooza that afternoon, went to work for the first time in five weeks on Monday (yes, it was strange, but also comforting), slept all day Tuesday (post-prednisone crash), got a cold/bronchitis/new antibiotics on Wednesday/Thursday, and my lockdown instructions this morning. No allergic itchiness, no extreme bony pain; just life, but with cancer/chemo.

A few days after my lockdown, my blood counts rebounded. Michael and I celebrated by leaving the apartment to run errands on a sunny weekend afternoon, and found ourselves at Whole Foods.

Since starting chemo, the carefully constructed diet I'd followed for the previous five years had gone completely out the window. No longer did I avoid gluten, cow dairy, pork, processed meats, and non-organic food. I had lost so much weight and, when I was hungry, was so absolutely ravenous that I ate anything, paying special tribute to the foods I deeply craved: salty, greasy, bready deliciousness. At the top of this list were barbeque, any noodle dish from any culture (especially pad thai and fettucine carbonara), and sandwiches.

Sandwiches, in my humble opinion, are God's gift to humanity. And when you choose to avoid gluten, eating sandwiches borders on the impossible because, let's be honest, gluten-free sandwich bread is terrible. So when you jump back into the land of gluten, a whole world of bread opens up to you: farmhouse rye, crunchy-yet-tender baguettes, focaccia, pretzel rolls, and the simple-yet-not-at-all-simple whole-grain sliced sandwich bread.

We found ourselves at Whole Foods not because we needed groceries, but because we needed lunch. I was at the point in my chemo cycle where I was starving all the time. On this day, I craved a true Italian hoagie. This particular breed of sandwich is not Chicago's strong suit, but the city valiantly tries and, for the most part, some delis succeed. One of those delis is the enormous Whole Foods a couple miles from our apartment.

In the parking lot, I put all my focus into my chemo-weakened muscles and sprinted to the deli counter. Not wishing to beat me there, Michael walked alongside me as slowly as he could.

"Italian on a baguette with extra everything, including *giardiniera*. Add mayo, and please don't skimp on the lettuce," I wheezed to the chef, fully winded from my three-minute, hundred-yard dash.

Giardiniera is a wonderful Italian invention adopted by Chicago as an essential food group. It's basically pickled peppers, and the most amazing sandwich topping ever—second only to mayonnaise, which has been my first food love for as long as I can remember. I never tried *giardiniera* before I got sick, because before I got sick, I hated spicy food. But for four days after every round of chemo, my mouth tasted like I spent all my free time licking aluminum foil, and spicy food was the only thing with any flavor. Luckily for my taste buds, this whole new world of flavors was something I continued to enjoy even after the metallic flavor disappeared from my palate. Suddenly, my old favorites were new again. Later, I figured out that spicy food triggered my hot flashes, but at this point I was having them all the time anyway, so bring on the *giardiniera*.

"Do you want anything to drink?" Michael asked, eying the salad bar behind him as the lovely woman at the deli constructed my processed meat monstrosity.

"Ginger beer!" I was delighted. Spicy soda! "I'll go get some."

"Okay, I'll make a salad. See you back here?" His eyes crinkled as he looked at me, love and concern etched across his furrowed brow. It took me longer than it should have to realize that the minute I started treatment, he worried about me whenever I was not in his line of sight—and probably even when I was.

"Yes, bear, I'll be back soon." I kissed his cheek and sprinted off. Two minutes later, I got to the soda aisle that was twenty feet away and started scanning the shelves for the ginger beer.

Ah! There it was, on the bottom shelf. I reached down, grabbed a four-pack, and stopped. I couldn't pick it up. The two or three pounds (if that) of glass and liquid had halted all upward progress.

Shit. Now what?

I clutched one of the shelves with my left hand and tried to pull myself up. No dice. I put the ginger beer on the ground, slowly straightened my back, and assessed the situation.

Well, my back is weak. So what. My legs are probably stronger.

I hatched a plan.

I crouched down into a squat, using the shelves to support my downward progress. With my butt near my heels, I picked up the four-pack again and started to straighten my legs. And stopped again.

I was stuck. I needed both hands to climb up the shelves to stand up, but I couldn't use both hands if I was holding the soda. I got out of the crouch and onto my hands and knees and tried again. And failed.

I sat down with my back to the shelves. I was bald and emaciated. Surely someone would help me up.

Are you fucking kidding me? I used to be a Division I college rower! I could bench-press my own weight! And now I can't pick up a GODDAMNED FOUR-PACK OF SODA*? It's not even a six-pack! What the fuckedy-fuck-fuck?*

I took a deep breath. After all, this was not an irretrievable situation. Michael would soon figure out where I was. He would come help me.

But I was so tired of being the weak link—of being sick even when I thought I was having a moment, just a moment, when I didn't have to be sick. Cancer was always there, reminding me that I wasn't me. And the worst part was that Michael never got a break from it either.

The least you can do is not get stuck on the floor at Whole Foods, Lydia.

I shut off that voice immediately, knowing that she tends to get me nowhere. I was still trapped, like a turtle that had been flipped onto its back. Tears started rolling down my cheeks. Was this really the point? Sure, these drugs might be killing the cancer, but at what cost?

Ever since starting chemotherapy, my body had become unrecognizable to me. My strong muscles had collapsed under the chemical attack. My slender, athletic frame had shrunk. I had started to curl in on myself, using my shoulders and back to protect my heart from its grapefruit-sized tumor and the toxic drugs. With that physical desecration, my self-confidence and inner faith had begun to waver. Ignoring my sister's advice, I started to question the decision to go through with it.

Why did this happen? Why did I agree to this course of treatment? What is happening to me? Will I ever get out of this? Will I ever GET OFF THIS FLOOR*?*

All I wanted was my absurd Dagwood and my spicy soda and a spot in the sun where I could consume all of it. Instead, I was sprawled on the floor, contemplating whether I had the strength to pull over the shelves of groceries and end my misery.

Michael found me a few moments later, a weepy, bald shell of the woman he married. "Um, why are you on the floor?"

"I couldn't stand up!" I was irate and crying and might have even slapped the floor in frustration.

He barked out a laugh and then stopped, and he then couldn't stop. "I'm sorry," he gasped, "but this is hilarious."

"NO, IT'S NOT!" I heaved. He and I looked at each other, his eyes dancing, mine fiery. With each surging breath, I felt the floor pushing against my butt bones and the shelf of glass bottles pushing into my spine and ribs. "Okay, maybe it is. A little bit."

He leaned over, picked up the soda, and pulled me up from the floor.

"I hate cancer," I grumbled, a small smile leaking onto my face.

"Yup. It sucks." He kissed my cheek, and I walked to the check-out line with my hand in his, propelled by my gratitude for not showing me the burden he carried. Maybe this was what partnership was about. And maybe I needed to cut myself some slack.

AFTER TWO ROUNDS of chemo, Dr. Levi announced that the PET scan showed "striking improvement," which meant the tumor itself was much less active—and 33 percent of its original size. Instead of a grapefruit, I had a tangerine.

After round four, the tumor shrank from 6 cm x 3 cm to 6 cm x 2 cm, and the PET scan could barely distinguish it from surrounding tissue. Radiology and oncology translated this information in a positive light: what remained of my tumor was dead. My chemo protocol insisted that I still needed to receive two rounds of R-EPOCH after "complete visual resolution," just to make sure. I was simply grateful that it would be finished after six rounds instead of the anticipated eight or the dreaded ten. Progress in a land with no maps is still progress.

I met this news with such delight that I immediately turned to my trusty iPad. As I began to blog about being cancer-free, though, I realized that everything I was experiencing had nothing to do with cancer and everything to do with chemotherapy. And then I got pissed off. And then I did a full inventory. And then I got more pissed off. And then I realized that I wouldn't be bitching about chemo if I still had cancer, so I calmed down a bit. But either way, the relief over being cancer-free (sort of) was overshadowed by the physical symptoms that I was managing, and would continue to manage, for two more rounds of chemotherapy—and who knew how long afterward.

After this mental gymnastics, I blogged:

I HAVE CHEMO!

Now that my various doctors have decided that my tumor is cancer-free and that I have twelve cubic centimeters of dead cells lodged in my chest, it's official! I no longer have cancer; I have chemo.

I'm bald, and I'm losing my eyebrows and eyelashes, too. Actually, by the time those are gone, the only hair I will have left on my body is my arm hair (I'm pretty sure

I've lost my nose hair too, which just makes me laugh). This is both fabulous and frustrating. I don't need to shave or wax or spend time blow drying my hair, which is amazing (although I was never accused of spending a tremendous amount of time doing any of that before). However, losing my eyebrows makes my face look blank, and losing my eyelashes has erased the natural definition around my eyes. I'm not a makeup person, but I've spent the last few weeks learning how to solve these problems—more or less successfully. Along those same lines, my nails have stopped growing, are weak, and have started peeling away in fine layers. Dr. Levi recommended nail polish to help keep them intact. So as my face has lost its definition, I'm making up for it with blue, green, and orange fingers and toes.

My skin feels like it's going to crumble and fall off. Dehydration is a natural side effect with chemo, and now that Chicago has entered "fall" (which really feels more like winter in other parts of the world), I'm contemplating taking lotion baths. The dehydration is a hard problem to solve because I get mouth sores, which makes drinking water painful. At the same time, my teeth have gotten ridiculously sensitive, so the only liquids I can drink have to be just about body temperature and even then only through a straw. I solve some of this problem by going to Dr. Levi's office every (weekday) morning when I'm not in the hospital to get an infusion of between one and two liters of fluid, but it's not a complete solution.

The tips of my fingers have been either tingling or numb for the last month and a half. This is a specific side effect caused by the drug vinchristine. It attacks the sheathing around the nerves, which starts to kill off the ability for the nerve to do its job. Fingers and toes are the first to go, because the nerves that feed them are the longest in the body. A drug called Neurontin helps contain the damage, but I'm constantly worried that my reflexes will be forever compromised.

I have dropped from a healthy 130 pounds for my five-foot-six frame to 110. The last time I saw that number on a scale was when I was fourteen years old. I have no fat reserves and no ability to control my own fluctuating temperature, let alone the hot flashes caused by my chemical (hopefully not permanent) menopause. These hot flashes go throughout the day, but get much worse at night. At night, I have a pile of T-shirts by the bed so I can change my shirt easily, and I also sleep on two towels. Right after chemo, I go through three shirts and both towels each night. After about a week, I'm down to one or two shirts with no towels.

As for being an athlete in a former life, I poke the big muscles in my legs, amazed at their level of atrophy. Muscle atrophy, for the most part, is caused by the chemotherapy but some of it does have to do with my own fatigue and inability to do some of the most basic things for at least 1.5 out of every 3 weeks. Like walking. I also noticed within the past two weeks that I can't really wear heels anymore because my little muscles in my legs aren't capable of stopping an ankle role or a trip up a curb. I can't even imagine what this will be like once I start trying to jog again. Speaking of jogging, I have shortness of breath—not like the kind I had when my tumor was sitting on my heart, but more like I've been breathing air in New York or Beijing for too long. It will get better as I exercise more, but right now, I can't swim a lap in a pool, walk up a flight of stairs, or jog more than a block without needing to stop and catch my breath.

Let's not forget neutropenia and all of the other lovely blood things! Just about five days after I get out of the hospital, my blood counts plummet. By plummet, I mean that I go from having a happy immune system filled with white blood cells to an incredibly unhappy immune system with some very lonely white blood cells wandering around in a sea of red blood cells and plasma. After four rounds of chemo, they don't even have platelets around to keep them company either, which just makes for sad blood. And a sad Lydia. I have to stay home and generally avoid contact with other people (germs, you know). Plus I start getting nose bleeds because of the platelet issue. So I'm wandering around my apartment with my cats, no immune system, a bloody tissue, and I can't even have sushi or unpasteurized cheese to make the whole thing more pleasant. And that's not all! During my hospital stay, the chemo kicks the crap out of my hemoglobin/red blood cells, so I have to have a blood transfusion there. Which is actually pretty great, because my energy drops along with the hemoglobin (it's hard for my blood to transport oxygen without hemoglobin), so the transfusion gives me a nice little boost. However, it's temporary because of the overall exhaustion associated with this entire delightful experience.

Last but not least is my dramatic fatigue. As chemo has gone on, I've simply gotten more and more tired. Some office colleagues asked what it was like, and I used an example that unfortunately most of them are fairly familiar with. After billing a 100-hour week (that's billing, mind you, which is usually about an hour or two less a day than actual working time, so a 100-hour billing week translates into being functional and in the office between 15–17 hours a day, seven days a week), you come home on Sunday night and sit on the couch and stare at the wall. That's how I feel ALL THE TIME. They both looked at me, appalled.

Is this better than cancer? Well, hopefully chemo won't kill me while cancer would. But wow, there must be a better solution. In the meantime, I have chemo instead of cancer. Am I thrilled about this? Talk to me when my hair starts growing back.

My last round of chemo was in late October, and I couldn't stop myself from kissing the door of my hospital room on my way out. When Michael appeared to pick me up and take me home, I collapsed into his arms under the weight of my relief and in gratitude for his unfailing support. Appreciation leaked out of every pore of my body—for my doctors and nurses and techs and parents and sister and cousins and friends who had all helped me get to the point where I could walk out of the hospital, using my own legs, with a small dead tumor in my chest.

Walk? I didn't walk. I floated. Down the hall, into the elevator, and out of the hospital—my feet never touched the ground. I didn't care that it took me longer than ever to get from one door to the next, from one intersection to the next. I didn't care that my breathing was more labored now. I simply floated home, holding hands with my person, grateful beyond measure to finally be done.

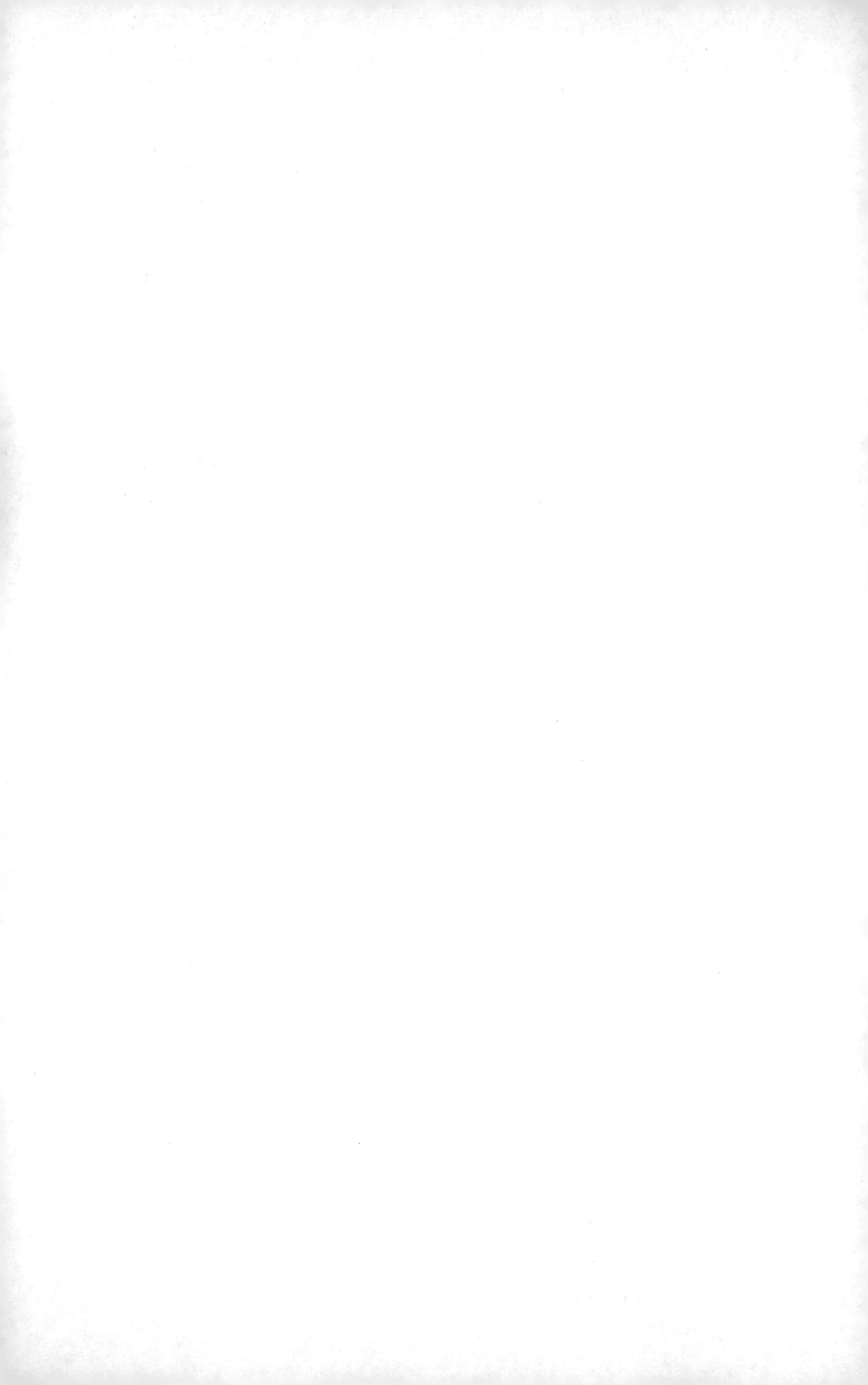

PURPOSE

WHEN I ARRIVED for my freshman year at Brown University in the fall of 1997, I reminded myself of the promise I had made the previous spring: *college has nothing to do with Michael*. In general, I kept this promise. For the first few months, I turned down a different path or sidewalk when I saw anyone on crutches. Eventually, when he was off crutches and could move away from me first, I stopped seeing him altogether.

I began to recover. I found a kind boy who reminded me of a blond high school soccer player I had known once upon a time. I found a supportive group of friends. I struggled with engineering classes and thrived in architectural history and political science. I drank too much on Thursday nights and gained the obligatory "freshman fifteen." In short, I shook myself off and began my next chapter.

I couldn't fully forget, though. Michael was there in my dreams. He was there when I closed my eyes. And sometimes, he was actually there in my email.

I've been going to therapy . . .

Maybe you should consider finding a therapist . . .

I'm sorry . . .

Finally, I caved to the memories and just showed up on his doorstep. The sight of him hit me like a freight train. How could I ever be with just a nice, smart guy, if this intensity was lying in wait around the corner? Months had passed since I'd last seen him, but there it was, simultaneously breathtaking, piercing—powerful enough to make me stagger—and calming, healing, soothing. A piece of me had gone missing, and his presence restored it. Violently.

On his doorstep that day, Michael seized me with similar force, and for thirty-six hours we lived in a bubble of our own creation. And then, knowing we couldn't work without a lot of therapy—and a lot of maturity, which neither of us had—we left each other. Again.

AS I MOVED from engineering to economics and finally to the delight of urban studies . . . from being an athlete to coaching middle-school athletics . . . from childhood to the beginnings of adulthood . . . the intensity of losing Michael eased. I fell in and out of love, but it was never the same. I chalked it up to "everything feels different when it's not the first," but I never quite believed that was the case.

After graduation in 2002, I moved first back to DC and then, a year later, to Boston, where I found a career helping the Commonwealth of Massachusetts manage its relationship with its cities and towns. For extra cash, I also tended bar at a dark den frequented by Harvard and MIT students. I reveled in routinely conversing with cute, brooding blonds who could sweep me off my feet with a clear-eyed look of remarkable intelligence, but I kept at a comfortable distance, as the physical barrier between patron and bartender remained impermeable no matter how much alcohol was consumed.

I was stretching my mind in a worthwhile career, stretching my social life after-hours. I was, in short, a yuppie in my twenties. And like so many yuppies in their twenties, I eventually found someone to marry.

Luke was lovely: kind, smart, attractive, and without the baggage of failed, dramatic young love. We laughed together all the time—something I was absolutely not used to in a partner, and something I discovered that I needed.

By January 2007, I had quit bartending and moved up enough in my career that I found myself working directly for senior leadership in the administration of Governor Deval Patrick, in an office with an enormous window that looked out over the Boston Common. My colleagues were smart and dedicated, and I loved my days in the statehouse brainstorming, negotiating, and writing on solutions for the sticky and fascinating problems faced by Massachusetts communities. Most of all, I loved working toward a purpose larger than myself.

This desire to devote myself to a purpose, to help in some significant way, has been present in me for as long as I can remember. Unlike those friends of mine who always knew exactly what they wanted to be when they grew up—fireman, lawyer, banker, parent, doctor, pilot, veterinarian—my desire never manifested in a particular career. I just wanted to help. So when friends fought, I brokered truces. I helped lost animals.

I coached sports. I looked to my parents and how their drive to help manifested in federal government administration, United Nations and UNESCO work, and teaching, and thought about how I, too, could contribute.

In DC I had worked in real estate, helping the built environment work better for the people who lived in dilapidated neighborhoods. In Boston, I had a broader mandate: to help the cities and towns empower their citizens to succeed, and to help the state make sure those communities thrived. Still, I wondered if I was doing enough. Could I do it at a higher level, and if so, how?

The answer was obvious: in my family, when we want to up the ante, our default is to go back to school.

I LANDED IN CHICAGO in August 2008 for Northwestern's JD-MBA program and was immediately astonished by how different my life became. Even the air there was different from on the East Coast; the lack of salt as I ran along the lakefront was palpable, changing the very way I breathed. I had to consciously inhale more deeply, making up with mental energy what my body did naturally when surrounded by salt air. And everyone was just too damn nice, from the clerk at CVS to the homeless man near my apartment to the salaried administrators at school. People in Chicago did not spend their time thinking long thoughts about the nature of humanity as they did in the home of the Boston Tea Party; they were too busy attending to the nuts and bolts of reality.

This worked well for me, because straightaway I was buried in my studies. For the first time in my life, I had to work absurdly hard to hold my own among my classmates. Everyone there had been a top college student at a top college somewhere in the world. This really was the best of the best of the best. On top of that, the courses were different from any I'd ever taken. Law school doesn't teach facts; it teaches a different approach. Every day, I would show up to a lesson on contracts or torts and feel as though my brain were being rewired. And the only way to achieve this rewiring was to engage with all of my effort—in the classroom, in my homework, and with my classmates and new friends.

It was exhausting. I was working so hard that I started losing weight again. The marathon I had been training for fell to the wayside, although the running did not. Disappearing down the lakeshore for an hour every day with music blasting in my ears was my only respite from the incessant demands on my creativity and intellect. Besides sleep, running was the only rest I could find.

And I loved it all. I thrived. I had never been stretched intellectually in such a way. The weird complications of the law, and the strange nuances of subtle argument and persuasive writing, fed me even as the difficulty drained me.

My relationship bore the brunt of my exhaustion. Luke was in graduate school himself, living in Michigan, facing all sorts of existential questions and leaning on me to help answer them. As my energy waned, I needed him to help fuel me but found that he only drained me further. Our conversations, previously light and funny and sweet, became heavier and more laden with complicated matters. His own growth was beginning to feel like yet another part of my workload, an assignment or problem I had to research, contemplate, and (ultimately) solve.

By early October, I was completely twisted apart, convinced that law school was killing my relationship—but afraid to talk about it. I would close the door to my apartment each day, leaving the boxes of unfinished wedding save-the-dates lying on the table, and return too drained to address the ten I'd budgeted for that evening. After a while, the ivory envelopes started to look accusatory, like fancy little lies in black calligraphy.

And then, in mid-October, Facebook pinged with a note from Michael.

I had joined Facebook six months previously and created my friendship group by scooping friends from friends. When I had reached Michael's name, I thought, *It's been almost ten years since we last had any kind of a conversation. Time enough for our past to be resolved. What could possibly go wrong?*

I clicked on his name.

After receiving the notification, he later told me, he spilled his water bottle and nearly fell out of his chair. He let it go for a few days, but I was constantly popping up on his screen. It got to the point where he couldn't let it continue without some kind of acknowledgment. So he sent me a quick note to say hi. Among the relevant life details: he was living in Chicago, working as chief technology officer for Barack Obama's 2008 presidential campaign.

I responded with equally factual words—I'm heading to Chicago to start law school, been working in government, glad that we both seem to be doing good work—and that was it. Until his name appeared on my screen again in early October, a few weeks before the election: How's being a student again? You liking Chicago—or too buried in your first year of school to see it yet?

I was so frayed that my usual mental barriers around all-things-Michael did not have a chance to activate. I recognized his name and knew he had nothing to do with the stress of my fiancé or the exhaustion of law school. So, I responded with some version of the truth about my life at that moment.

A few notes later, we determined that eating a burger at a place I hadn't yet tried would be a nice way to pull both of us out of our respective tornados, if just for a moment. He was trying to stay functioning through the end of the campaign; I was trying to stay focused on what could nurture me through the end of the first semester.

Dinner was strange.

Physically, Michael was different. His blond hair was darker. His skin was gray. He was simultaneously bigger than I remembered and also weirdly emaciated. His voice, always deep, had become gravelly, and he had the jumpy demeanor of someone who had been living on coffee and cigarettes for far too long. In short, he looked like hell.

"Jesus Christ, what happened to you?" I couldn't help but blurt out after we first greeted each other and completed a carefully negotiated hug.

"Two years of a presidential campaign," he replied. "I was at the clinic today with heart palpitations. They told me I had to quit either coffee or cigarettes. I quit coffee."

I shrugged. "Well, that's not that big of a deal."

"It is when you're drinking twenty-five shots of espresso a day."

He was still stubborn. And intense.

I changed the subject. We were at dinner to acknowledge each other's presence after ten years of radio silence. But Michael also had questions—about what it was like to work in government, how it was different from a campaign, and so forth. He asked about Luke; I asked about his girlfriend. I noticed that he wasn't eating his food. I asked if there was anything on his mind that prompted his reaching out to me.

He put his fork down as if in preparation for something serious, which I found amusing. It was such a cliché. He took a deep breath and looked at me with clear eyes. "I wanted to apologize for my behavior ten years ago, and to give you the opportunity to ask me any questions you may have about what happened."

I sat back. I had not expected this. I also had not expected to see his eyes so calm. He was in the middle of a maelstrom at work, and his body was shutting down, but his eyes were clearer than I had ever seen them. He wasn't just different physically. The previous ten years seemed to have shifted something deep inside him.

He kept talking: "You were the best part of my life back then, and I never meant for you to get hurt. I'm sorry."

For so many years after we left each other, I had played out this conversation in my head. It usually involved me shouting at him and then kicking him in the crotch. It had never started with him calmly apologizing and opening the door to dialogue. I hadn't had any kind of thought about this or him in a long time. Now that it was happening, the desire to shout and rage and hurt him had passed. I was pleasantly surprised to notice this.

The apology did soothe some hidden rough edge of my psyche, though, and the curiosity remained. "Well, since you mentioned it, would you mind sharing what actually happened? It was a, um"—I searched for the right word—"confusing time for me."

The story that unfolded began to clear up many of my

lingering questions about that period in my personal history. The lies, the cheating, the pain. The feeling that we couldn't shake each other. The avalanche of emotions that I felt whenever I saw him or heard his voice. Puzzle pieces in my mind, out of place for so long, clicked. My body relaxed in a long-forgotten way.

Then we realized that we had been at dinner for four hours, and both of us still had work to do that night. As we quickly gathered up our coats and left the restaurant, he chuckled to himself. "I haven't stepped away from my office or my phone for four hours in the past two years, except to sleep."

I felt guilty. "I'm sorry!"

"I knew what I was doing." He smiled. "Don't take responsibility for something that isn't yours."

I was thunderstruck. I didn't know if he meant for those words to apply to more than just those four hours, but my brain and my battered sense of self construed them in the most expansive way possible.

For years I had blamed myself for Michael's disappearing act. *If only I could have helped. If only I had done something different. If only I hadn't been such a useless girlfriend . . .* In the wake of that destructive time, I had subtly changed my behavior. I'd stopped having complete faith in my ability to read people. I'd stopped feeling proud of my ability to help friends see a chaotic moment from another perspective. I'd stopped feeling as though I possessed insight and emotional intelligence.

Although therapists and friends and family had given me this same message for years—*not your responsibility, not your responsibility*—I had never really believed it. Now here *he* was, the instigator of this whole mess, telling me the same thing: it wasn't my responsibility. Hearing it from him now gave me the opportunity to forgive myself. To reopen the doors to a side of my personality that I had closed off.

We hugged again, both glad for the small, simple fact that we were less uncomfortable with each other.

I left that night feeling as though I had done what I needed to do. Now I could get back to my impending marriage—and hundreds of pages of reading. Yet I still harbored a latent curiosity. Michael's explanation of things had answered some questions but inevitably brought more to the surface. Given how fundamentally our relationship—and the destruction of said relationship—had impacted me, I wanted to understand it. Especially with respect to what was happening in my current relationship. If I was still reacting to old problems, I wanted to clean them up before I pledged myself, for life, to Luke. And given my newfound love of the law and the ways it was teaching me to look at a problem, I wanted to examine this from every angle.

For the next two weeks, Michael and I emailed each other questions and thoughts and answers. School kept asking the most out of me. My relationship kept pulling on me. I found myself taking solace not just in sleep and running, but in the words that emerged from my inbox once or twice a day. I soon became aware what was going on: I was wading through muddy waters.

It was time to find a therapist.

HALF OF WHAT law schools do these days is make sure their students are not losing their minds. After several brief conversations with professors I had learned to trust, I found Ruth, my no-holds-barred therapist. I laid my confusion at her feet, like a penitent begging for guidance. Or answers. Or something. Anything, really.

Ruth saw immediately that I spent all my time in my head, and that my brain was not going to help me out of this mess. And she began the process of teaching me that my body, too, has wisdom. For the first time in my adult life, I started down the road of learning to appreciate that body wisdom is just as powerful as mind wisdom. What's more, body wisdom is always honest.

At first, I didn't know how to ignore my brain long enough to let the messages from my body leak through to awareness. But Ruth was trained and practiced, and she could discern when my brain got in the way. With great patience, she helped me work through the increasing frustration at my failure to immediately grasp my body's intuition and the wisdom I had spent years ignoring.

"Do you like law school?"

My gut tweaked in happiness. My brain's voice yelped in confusion. "I don't know."

"That's not true," Ruth countered. "A small smile appeared on your face before your brain jumped in. What did you feel when I asked you that question?"

I didn't really know how I felt, because my brain instantly got in the way with all of its questions. "My gut clenched with . . . excitement, maybe?"

"Okay, let's try it again. Clear your mind. Take a long breath in. One . . . two . . . three . . . four. Hold it. And now let it out. One . . . two . . . three . . . four. Drop your shoulders. Relax."

With Ruth's guidance, I began to learn how to relax my body and quiet my brain. I practiced and practiced until, when she asked me a question, I could actually feel my instinctual answer. This took weeks.

Meanwhile, school continued to get harder, more demanding. My relationship with Luke continued to get more and more frustrating. Michael's emails, which landed in my inbox once or twice a day, left me utterly confused.

At some point in early December, I realized that Michael and I had cleaned up the past and were now leaning on each other for support in the present. I was studying for exams; he was in DC, working on transitioning the new administration, as busy as ever. And while we were busy leaning on each other, my fiancé was still relying on me.

One day at therapy, after months of training my mind to be nice and quiet—long enough, at least, for me to recognize the wisdom of my body's reactions—Ruth finally dropped the question: "What would happen if you broke it off with Luke?"

My body flooded with relief, my shoulders relaxed, and my head came up. I took a deep breath of quiet gratitude.

"What would happen if you stopped speaking to Michael?"

My body clenched in agony, my shoulders crumbled under an unseen weight, and a small sob leaked from my mouth.

OH. SHIT.

Ruth sat back in her chair. "Well, I think you have your answer."

THE LAST DAY of the semester, I took my property exam in the morning and broke off my engagement in the afternoon. Half an hour into the conversation, it became clear that Luke also did not want to get married, and we ended up talking for two hours with a lightness that neither of us had felt in each other's presence for months. Together, we drafted an email to our family and friends, explaining that they no longer had to save the date for our wedding. Then we hugged and said good-bye before Luke drove back to Michigan.

"I'm proud of you," Ruth said after hearing my triumphant tale. "Now, have a wonderful holiday."

I opened a bottle of bourbon, ordered a pizza, and didn't leave my apartment for three days. I reread emails from Michael, watched almost every season of *Alias* in the DVD box set, and realized that I had fallen back in love with my ex-boyfriend from hell. He had been fairly straightforward about his feelings for me for a couple of weeks—and had been patiently waiting for me to figure myself out.

Two months later, Michael left DC, returned to Chicago, and moved into my apartment. We didn't get married right away for a few reasons. We had to give my side of the aisle time to wrap their heads around the scenario—the fact that I didn't just swap one guy for another, even though the new (old) guy showed up fairly quickly. Also, my family and friends had last seen Michael, for the most part, as the nineteen-year-old who broke my heart. Some bridges needed reconstructing. Finally, Michael himself needed to recover from his serious case of "campaign." Every day, I would wake up and head to school. He would wake up in time to make and bring me lunch. Then he would exercise (haltingly at first) and work on the small consulting project that occupied two to three hours of his day. Then he would make dinner and head back to bed. It took him months of self-care to return to full strength.

At one point in the middle of this recovery, I looked at him and asked why he allowed himself to get so drained. He thought about it for a minute, and then responded, "Because I owe them."

"Owe who?" I asked.

"Them." He waved his hand around in a circle, indicating simultaneously everyone and no one. "I need to make sure my life is useful."

I took a deep breath. This part of Michael was new. Although I was impressed with his commitment, what he was willing to go through for it made me anxious.

As the weeks passed, his hair lightened, the stress fell from his shoulders, his cheeks colored, and he quit smoking. In early May, on a beautiful spring day, he asked me to be his forever. I jokingly qualified my yes with one caveat: no more campaigns. He laughed in agreement.

We married a year later in a California vineyard under the clear blue sky. It was, we agreed, the only thing big enough to contain what we felt for each other. As we'd both learned, nothing short of our own idiocy could keep us apart.

MARRIAGE

THE HONEYMOON PHASE of our marriage lasted exactly eight months, from the day of our wedding until the night Michael told me he wanted to rescind his promise and join the 2012 Obama reelection campaign. I remember the exact moment: how I sat in our bed, my hand paused on its way to turn off the light. How I pulled my legs into my belly and felt the bottom drop out of my world. *He must be joking*, I thought. The last campaign had almost killed him.

"Could you say that again, please?" I managed once I found my voice. He had promised me that there would be no more.

I still don't remember his exact response. Something about hope and change, about wanting to ensure Obama got a second term. Something about being needed on the campaign, making sure it had a heart. Something about a bunch of bullshit, as far as I was concerned. I was fully convinced that President Obama would win with or without Michael. My husband's wounds from the 2008 campaign were still too raw. At least for me.

"Um, are you really telling me that the sitting president of the United States *needs* you to be on his campaign in order to win? No offense, but that takes your usual arrogance to a whole new level."

Michael seemed sure this time around would be different.

I snorted—actually snorted. "Are they asking you to be campaign manager? Because unless they are, there's not a chance in hell this one will be truly different." I made it clear that I wasn't remotely comfortable with this decision. "And you're going to have to do a hell of a lot to prove to me otherwise."

Major rule of any relationship, as any loving couple knows: never go to bed angry. For the first time in our marriage, I broke that rule. I turned off the light and rolled away from my husband, that night and for months afterward.

I refused to believe that his choice of career was worth the damage it would do to him, and I desperately wanted to protect him from that choice. But I didn't choose the best way to go about it. I have no idea what my plan was—be furious with him, day after day, night after night, until he just changed his mind? God knows what I was thinking! Once my husband sets out on a path, only something tremendous will deter him from it.

Predictably, the campaign was terribly demanding in the way that all campaigns are. And instead of causing any real change, I abandoned Michael right when he needed my support the most. Oops. He would slog to work under a cloud of his wife's fury and then slog home to an unsympathetic ear. I did try to help him think through some of the problems, but all under the burdensome veil of my opinion that he'd made his bed and should learn to sleep in it.

If only I had seen how unhelpful and undermining my

approach was. If only Michael had responded with something useful, such as, *Could you please just accept my choice and support me?* or *Perhaps we should go to marital therapy to work through it,* or even *Wow, you're really dead set on being a nightmare during this.* Instead, he just started getting quieter about everything: his job, his emotions, his thoughts . . . and our marriage.

IN THE LAST semester of my joint program, I was working part-time for the general counsel of the Clinton Foundation, doing the work I came to law school to do: helping for-purpose organizations succeed. I was also taking courses like administrative law, a class that I loved—much to the bafflement of my classmates and, in some respects, the professor. The coursework reminded me how much I thrived on the intricacies of large government institutions.

I found a number of things about this course stimulating: the skill it takes to get a law to the point where it impacts an actual person; the nuance of law versus regulation versus rule; the complex nature of what it takes to be a government of the people, by the people, and for the people—when all 325 million of those people are completely different. In short, administrative law brought me back to why I went to law school in the first place. I wasn't there to have my brains scrambled; that was simply an entertaining by-product. I was there to make myself a more skilled citizen of the world, to hone my desire to help in some specific way.

For the entire three years of my program, I had been thinking about what my job would be after graduating. Being creative in this search is difficult, because law schools are designed around feeding students into law firms, and business schools are designed around feeding students into investment banks, consulting firms, or Fortune 500 companies. I resisted on-campus recruiting at first, but as I spent more time tending my fragile marriage, I didn't have the time to be creative, so I succumbed to on-campus recruiting. In the end, I landed a great job offer in public-sector consulting, at IBM's offices in Washington, DC.

I had other options, too. The newly established Consumer Financial Protection Bureau had been courting me. I was a finalist for the Presidential Management Fellows program, which put me on the radar of the Justice Department, the White House, and the Office of Management and Budget. In short, my background combined with my current interests and education could launch me into any number of important and interesting jobs. It seemed clear that my next step would be working in or around the federal government, doing what I really wanted to do—and what I felt uniquely qualified, even called on, to do—with my skills and interests.

Michael's decision to return to the Obama campaign, which was based in Chicago, prompted a vital decision for me: Go to DC, and work for IBM or one of those other options? Or somehow come up with a job in Chicago, a year later than most students from my program had locked down their future after facing such decisions? It was 2011, three months before graduation, and I had no idea what to do.

I took this challenge home to Michael, who refused to state an opinion, knowing that it would sway my decision. So I sat with it for a while, weighing my desire to stay physically present in my tense marriage versus my desire to create change in the world. My professional future rested in one hand and our damaged little bird of a marriage in my other. The longer I sat with this choice, the more furious I became.

Michael had signed up for round two of the presidential campaign for no good reason, as far as I could tell. Yes, he too wanted to serve, but he could have done so in any number of ways, and he had chosen this particular one with no regard for the impact on us. As a result, I felt forced to consider taking a step back from launching my own career in the direction that I wanted. If we had actually sat down and thought through both career decisions at the same time, surely we could have figured out a way to serve our mutual goals in the same city. But his unilateral decision had cut off that option.

I sat down with my administrative law professor and laid my problem on his desk. He agreed that to do exactly what I wanted to do—my ideal job—I would have to leave Chicago. Furthermore, because it was so late in the recruiting process, I didn't have as much freedom to be creative about my options. Staying in Chicago would mean being less picky.

He looked at me. "If I can find you a job at a Chicago law firm, in something resembling your interests and skills, would you take it?"

I looked at him and heaved a sigh, resigned to the choice I was making, but also grateful for the offer on the table. "Yes."

"Great. Send me your résumé, and I'll see what I can do."

"Seriously? Just like that?" I was astounded. "Why is recruiting so complicated if you can just pull a job for me out of your email?"

"Because we're lawyers, and we like to complicate things unnecessarily." He was kidding, but behind his words lay a nugget of truth.

I had come to believe that if I made that same choice Michael had—putting my own personal desires above the concerns of the marriage—it would destroy our life together. So I reached a conclusion: if he wouldn't do what was necessary for the marriage, then I would.

I took a deep breath, swallowed my professional desires, and announced to my husband that if I could find a job in Chicago, I would stay. Yet Michael wasn't grateful. In fact, he seemed downright apathetic. I had chosen our marriage over my own professional opportunities, and I felt as though he was—if anything—disappointed in me. And I was furious.

My professor did as promised, and I received a job offer shortly after graduation, in corporate reorganization and bankruptcy law. Maybe I was taking my career backward instead of forward, but it was the only way I could see how to stay in Chicago. Perversely, my misgivings made me more committed to making my job work. I was determined to prove that my choice to stay in Chicago and save my marriage was the right one.

WORKING AS A practicing attorney could not have been more different from law school. Gone were the lofty mind-twisters, and in their place were office politics, research and drafting, and no small measure of basic administrative work. It was old in that it reminded me of my past working life, which I loved and missed, but it was new in every other way. I was tired from the long hours—and from the perplexing situation at home—but exhilarated to be working again with smart, interesting, and unexpectedly funny people.

More than anything, I was surprised by the fact that although I wasn't doing what I considered meaningful work, I still enjoyed it. I enjoyed the intellectual and legal challenges of my corporate clients (while happily ignoring many of the real-world ramifications of their actions), delighting in the new mental hurdles that I had to leap. It shocked Michael, too, who started making remarks along the lines of "I didn't think you would enjoy a job like this." To which I would respond, "Well, if you hadn't chosen to martyr yourself for the campaign, I wouldn't have taken a job like this in the first place."

I stayed angry. Meanwhile, Michael's initial quietness practically turned into mutism. Answers to "How was your day?" were answered with a flat "Fine." He spent more time watching TV and less time talking to me.

One freezing December morning as we walked hand in hand across the Wabash Avenue Bridge to work, I asked the question that brought everything to the surface: "Why aren't we having sex anymore?"

Michael didn't answer right away. I waited, with no clue what the answer would entail. We reached the intersection where usually we would turn our separate ways and head to work. This time, he turned to look at me instead. Searching my face with his hazel eyes, veiled against some emotion that I couldn't read on his face, he dropped my hand and pushed his hair away from his forehead.

"It's because home isn't comforting to me anymore," he said.

"You're not comforting to me anymore. Home doesn't feel like a refuge anymore. I'm going to spend a couple of days in a hotel."

And with that, he turned and walked away from me.

I was flabbergasted. Sure, the past few months had been hard, and we had been hard on each other as a result. But he had given no sign that this was where his mind had been heading.

"Wait!" I called after him. "You can't just drop that in the middle of the road and then walk away!"

He stopped walking, and I covered the distance in a few short seconds.

Clutching at his hand, I spun him around. "What the hell are you talking about? You can't just say you're miserable and then leave without talking to me about it!"

He pulled his hand out of my grip while simultaneously getting closer to me. "Stop shouting," he said in his quiet bass voice. "This isn't anyone's business but our own."

This seemed like a ludicrous response. Who gives a shit about a few angry words a bunch of random people overhear at 7:30 on a gray, freezing morning as they're heading to work? I said as much, but we were getting off track.

I took a deep breath. "You're so miserable that you can't even stay at home and talk to me about this tonight?"

"Yes."

"You didn't think to talk to me about it before it got this terrible?"

He just looked at me.

I had no idea what to do other than stand on that frozen Chicago corner, watching as the love of my life walked away from me once more.

AFTER THREE DAYS in a hotel, Michael came home. The rest of the winter and spring were pure hell.

My health was starting to deteriorate, but I was too distracted by relationship woes to pay much attention. By March 2012, I couldn't find solace even in my routine jog that had been keeping me sane during this painful time. At first, I would become winded after just a few miles. Then I could barely run a mile, and then just a few blocks would knock me for a loop. By April, I had a weird pain in my chest. Michael insisted that I go to the doctor, who diagnosed me with a pulled muscle and sent me home with Advil. Michael wasn't convinced, but I dug in, insisting that an X-ray was a waste of medical resources. The disagreement devolved into an argument by default, adding to the general discord.

In May, he moved out again, this time into a furnished one-bedroom apartment a few blocks away. I started losing weight. As I became more stressed, increasingly exhausted, and skinnier, I grew less and less inclined to deal with Michael's "crazy." I missed him as a person, but if this is what marriage with him would be like—everyone sacrificing their own desires for some larger, unknown plan—then forget it. My retorts became commensurately sharper. My awareness of what I wanted sharpened too. And my desire to keep him above all else began to fade.

Ruth had come back into my life, this time as a marital therapist. After some time learning how to communicate with each other in the confines of her office, my husband and I learned a few things. One, I was furious, utterly furious, about having to choose between our marriage or my career, when he very clearly didn't prioritize our marriage at all. Two, he was no longer convinced we were meant for each other, because if we were, then I should have been able to read his mind and realize how upset and alone he felt. Three, he felt that his own happiness—in his life, his marriage, his career—was less important than the impact he could make in the world.

Learning that *mind reader* was a marriage requirement left me flabbergasted. Learning that my husband's job was more important to him than our relationship left me feeling completely abandoned.

Gradually, other things started leaking in around the edges. The fact that I was enjoying my corporate job meant I wasn't the person he thought he'd married. My job, the only thing bringing me pleasure during those empty months, had become a refuge for me. I wasn't about to desert my only refuge, so I walled off my emotions about the problem and staunchly defended my work.

Meanwhile, Michael developed a new set of friends. When I was introduced, many of them struck me as the worst examples of life in the technology world: young, self-important douchebags.

As I changed in his eyes, he began to change in mine. Bizarrely, though, as we drifted further and further apart—to the point where we couldn't even converse without getting into a massive argument about how each had disappointed the other—I started rediscovering a side of my personality that I hadn't accessed for a long time. I stopped walking on eggshells around this martyr who had invaded my husband's body. I stopped listening to his increasingly outrageous accusations and pronouncements about my desires, my wishes, my character. I threw myself into work, where I was succeeding brilliantly. As much as I missed my marriage, I basically gave up on whether he liked me anymore.

So when his grandmother died and he insisted on going to the funeral alone, I told him to go fuck himself. As his wife, it was my obligation and desire to support his immediate family. When he would start in on me about my job or how I'd changed, I would cut him off and inform him, flatly, that whoever he had imagined he was marrying, this had always been the reality. I was still the same person I'd always been.

Some of the most absurd conversations focused on our nonexistent progeny. Suddenly, having kids was the most important thing to him, while it was the furthest thing from my mind. We were barely speaking to each other and hadn't had sex in months, yet Michael was insisting that if I didn't want children, that was a deal breaker. Ruth tried to introduce the idea that perhaps, with us feeling so distant from each other, neither was going to feel particularly strongly about having children.

He ignored her. When he stared at me, the walls behind his eyes were obvious. "So, do you want kids?"

I threw up my hands in frustration. "Absolutely not right now!"

He rolled his eyes. "Of course not now. I'm asking if you ever want kids. Do you ever want kids?"

Something in his face went beyond the question that was demanding an answer, but I didn't know what he was truly asking, and I didn't have the patience to try to unpack it. So I stayed with the topic at hand. "I have no idea. Are you ever going to stop acting like a crazy person?"

"I'll stop acting like a crazy person when you show me you're the person I married who wanted kids." He sat back, crossed his arms, and turned his face away from me, waiting for a miracle.

I answered the side of his face. "I don't want kids as long as our marriage is like this!"

"But once our marriage isn't like this, will you want kids?" He was looking at Ruth, who was letting the conversation go. I wondered if she saw the tiny ray of hope that passed over my face when he said *once our marriage isn't like this*.

I stopped to think about it. "When will that happen?" I quietly asked, genuinely curious to hear his answer.

"When you decide that you want kids."

Jesus Christ. "So our marriage will miraculously get better when I decide I want kids?"

"Yes."

"Great. Then I want kids." I can be a total pain in the ass sometimes.

"When?"

"Right now. Let's declare our marriage healed and have sex right now on this couch in Ruth's office so we can have kids."

Ruth, her face impassive, interrupted before our intellects would get us into any more trouble. My hope flickered out.

BY MID-JUNE, I couldn't even scurry across the street without completely losing my breath. One weekend, I couldn't keep any food down. I started waking up in the middle of the night with drenching night sweats, grateful that Michael wasn't in our king-sized bed so I could simply move to the dry side and fall back to sleep.

Although Michael and I were living apart, we started seeing each other once a week for a "date." After a few attempts at walking through the minefield, these rendezvous actually began to be fun. I would downplay my physical discomforts, chalking them up to the stress of our relationship, not wanting them to become a flashpoint. We would talk about current events and, tentatively, about each other's jobs. He seemed less insistent that the campaign was a good idea; I was too tired to extoll the virtues of corporate law. We both came away from our hard lines and started finding the joy in each other's presence again.

We had been falling apart for months, both holding on to our self-righteous anger. Since being physically separated, though, my anger had started to dissipate as I realized how much of my life it had consumed: my love for my brilliant, compassionate husband . . . my kindness toward my life partner . . . my own sense of strength . . . my desire to do more with my professional time. After four or five dates in as many weeks, we were coming slowly toward each other, drawn away from our corners of the boxing ring by the magnet within each of us that called to the other. We were quieter, calmer, more tender. We were able to see each other with more clarity and less emotion.

On Sunday, June 24, a few days before my next date with Michael, I went to brunch with my friend Elizabeth and then to yoga class by myself. Because I hadn't felt like myself for so long, I was barely phased when I woke that morning with a considerably swollen face. I figured that exhaustion explained the bags under my eyes and my swollen cheeks. Elizabeth saw something else, and she regarded me with genuine kindness and concern.

I explained it away with a wave of my hand and a quiet chuckle: "Stress."

As I moved into downward dog that afternoon, my cheeks throbbed and my eyes felt squashed. My hands were so puffy that my wedding ring was swallowed by skin. I picked my head up and the pressure lessened as I gazed at myself in the giant mirror. Dark, bloated circles under my eyes made them look smaller than usual. My mouth and nose seemed to disappear beneath splotchy, red, bulging cheeks. Even my neck seemed wider than usual.

I sat back onto my knees and kept looking in the mirror. Under the redness, my skin was pale. My shoulders had lost their muscular definition, and my collarbones were hidden. My arms resembled sausages. Yet my waist was much narrower than usual; I'd lost ten pounds in the past month, and the stretchy fabric of my size small yoga pants had plenty of room to spare.

I got up in the middle of class and left. I wandered home in a daze, took an Epsom salt bath in an effort to reduce the swelling, and stared at the wall for the rest of the night, holding Ellie as Jake purred against my thigh. The next day, I made an appointment to see my doctor that Thursday.

On my date with Michael, I didn't mention my impending appointment. We were busy trying to figure out logistics for that weekend. A friend of his was getting married in New York, and we hadn't yet figured out if I would join him at the black-tie wedding. As we were walking after dinner, he reached over and took my hand, laughing at something I'd said. "Okay," he conceded, "I'll take you as my plus-one."

"Your *plus-one*?" I shouted. "Fuck you! I'm your goddamn

wife!" But once the fury was spent, I was consumed with a wave of emotional weariness and started laughing.

Michael, chuckling, pulled me into a kiss.

The next morning, we were back on Ruth's couch, and Michael said he wanted to discuss something. He shared that a friend of his, upon hearing about what was going on with us, had given him a piece of advice: *If you want to be in the marriage, go home and be in the marriage. Talk to her. Be present. Otherwise, it sounds like you're just in a slow death spiral.*

I held my breath, wondering what Michael wanted to say.

He looked first at Ruth and then at me, picking up my hand from the couch. "I'd like to be in this marriage."

I burst into tears, simultaneously relieved and deeply afraid of how we were going to pick up the pieces.

Ruth let me weep while Michael held my hand. Then she asked, "When do you want to start being in your marriage?"

"Right now," he said. That night, we walked his clothing and toothbrush the few short blocks back to our life.

And then it was Thursday, June 28, 2012. That morning, I woke up next to Michael for the first time in two months. He looked at me, appalled, and said, "Is your face always this swollen in the morning?"

"I'm seeing my doctor at eleven. I'm sure it's nothing."

We got dressed and walked to work, hand in hand.

BACKWARD

SHORTLY AFTER FINISHING chemo, in late October 2012, Michael and I found ourselves back at home after four months of moving through a myopic tunnel of grief and terror. We no longer had the hospital to distract us from the state of our marriage. Our emotions were all over the place: Ecstatic to be done with chemo. Nervous about whether it completely worked. Excited that we weren't fighting anymore. Relieved that our relationship was paramount in our lives, as was now exceptionally obvious to both of us. But now what?

The tunnel—our hospital purgatory—had twisted and turned and spit us out somewhere unknown, somewhere different from that moment in June when our marriage was finally on the road back to health but everything else had suddenly gone to shit. Our job now was to remember that we were somewhere new, and to explore it in that way. It was time to find some grace in that new reality—not what we regretted or hoped, but what *was*. We had to discard old perspectives, old wounds and fights and triggers. We were new. We had a fresh opportunity to discover it together—to go for long walks, share ice cream sundaes, not talk too much, and promise each other to stay present.

Our human brains have the amazing ability to apply the lessons of the past to the future. As a result, they literally cannot stay in the present. The minute our brain observes something and reports it, that moment has already passed. So for me, the trick to staying present is simply to learn how to quiet the brain often enough that I can enjoy, say, the soft weight of Jake purring up against my thigh, without my brain commenting on how loud he is, how he needs to lose weight, how beautifully soft his fur is, how weird it is that these furry wildish animals run our household, blah blah blah.

Staying present is hard. And in that time after the hospital, it was not the first thought but the last resort. Michael and I had gone through so much to get to that quiet, calm, lovely ice cream sundae. Staying present seemed like the only way to handle this new stage of our relationship.

But everything else in the present? None of that seemed quite so precarious or precious. I was physically uncomfortable, mentally in agony, emotionally in distress, and spiritually unaware. Inside this swirl of massive discomfort, my higher functioning locked down and my limbic system activated. Short of a heroin trip (trust me, I contemplated it, but I've known too many who've fallen down that path), I couldn't flee my own body and my own mind. My only option, I thought, was to do what I always did: get on with the business of living.

When I'd heard the word *cancer* that June evening, my life as I knew it ended. Did it really end that very night? Of course not. My cancer had spent months growing, my body had spent months deteriorating, and I was sick in a thousand different ways before that doctor said *lymphoma*. But that's hard to remember when suddenly feeling crummy turns into *cancer* and *chemotherapy* and lots and lots of time in a hospital. So I emerged from the hospital in late October feeling as though my body and life had been ripped away from me four months earlier in a single stroke. And I decided to fight. I determined to get my life back as soon as humanly possible, come hell or high water.

Because the future was unknown, and the present was agonizing, I decided that the only way out was to go back to what I knew. Job. Body. Health, or my former concept of it.

This instinct echoed in the advice all around me:

Go back to work.

Go back to the gym.

Go back to your life.

Go back . . .

Go back . . .

Go back . . .

No one ever grabbed me by the shoulders and said, "Go forward." So, while I focused on the present of my marriage, I pressed my brain and my body backward into the only place that I knew: the past.

THREE DAYS AFTER I finished chemo for the last time, I walked into Dr. Levi's office to get my postchemo dose of fluids and shots.

"This is the last time I'll get fluids three days after chemo!" I announced to my nurse in sheer delight as she accessed my port, laughing. "When will I start feeling like myself again?"

She paused. "It depends on all sorts of things. But you'll stop feeling exhausted in about three months; and then in six months, you'll find it hard to believe that you thought you weren't exhausted at three months."

I can beat that, I thought smugly.

Three weeks out from chemo, Michael and I celebrated the end of two agonizing (and agonizingly long) milestones—his second Obama campaign and my chemotherapy—by getting on a plane to Los Angeles for a weekend in the sun. While there, we went for a two-hour hike, and I had to stop every few feet to let my heart catch up with my feet. And then I came home with a cold. Dr. Levi glared at me as she wrote out a prescription for antibiotics.

Five weeks out from chemo, I traveled again and came home with the flu. This time, Dr. Levi did more than glare as she handed over another prescription. "I get it. You've been pent up for months, and you're excited to be done. But your body is still really weak. Please, stop pushing it. No flights and no serious exercise for at least a month." And she signed the letter I had drafted to United Airlines explaining why I needed a flight change fee refund for a Miami wedding that weekend.

Two weeks later, we went to Italy. But I listened to Dr. Levi's advice. Seriously, I did. Between a long walk with Michael in the morning and a long walk in the evening while Michael worked, I would eat delicious food and sit quietly in a café and write, and then take a long nap. I slept ten hours a night. I sat back and allowed the people and culture and food of Italy to heal me. Bernini sculptures in Rome . . . the reddest tomatoes and freshest mozzarella on the thinnest pizza in Naples . . . a singing gondolier in Venice . . . and everywhere we turned, an ancient building or some adventure to be had at the end of a tiny alley. Michael gave me Neupogen shots at both airports: Chicago's O'Hare International and Milan's Malpensa. I didn't get sick. In fact, I came home feeling rested.

In December 2012, two months after finishing chemo, I could regularly stay up past 7 p.m. and hadn't pushed myself to the point of illness in at least a week. I declared myself "healed" and tentatively scheduled my return to work for the end of January—three months after chemo ended.

My latest CT scan (the 3-D X-ray) showed continued shrinkage of the tumor—now 25 percent of the original size. That was the good news. The PET scan, however, was lighting up in an unexpected way. Cancer cells love sugar, so they get very excited during the PET scan. The test shows how active organs and cells are after they absorb radioactive glucose. Mine should have shown less activity—none, ideally. This made no sense to me. It threw my newly found, carefully calibrated sense of calm into a state of panic and turmoil.

Dr. Levi described to me how my tumor was intricately wrapped around, wound through, or otherwise married to an organ in my chest called the thymus—a piece of information that was unnecessary for me to know until this moment. Who knew? I hated that I kept learning new things about my disease after it was supposed to be gone. My plans to go back to normal life came crashing all around me.

Dr. Levi wanted to remove the organ and my tumor to see what was going on. Sometimes it truly is cancer, but sometimes the thymus gland just gets pissed off at chemo and lights up a

PET scan. Short of pulling the whole thing out and looking at it under lots of microscopes, it's difficult to tell the difference. This sounded to me like a lot more hospital time, but she assured me that it could be done as outpatient surgery, and sent me off to meet Dr. McLean, my new thoracic surgeon.

Dr. McLean swept into the room trailing medical students and residents, an entourage befitting the head of the department but not his personality. The penitents faded into the background as he sat down with me, gently held my hands, and carefully made the case for opening up my chest in order to capture the entirety of the tumor. He explained that if he pulled out only bits and pieces of the tumor in a less invasive procedure, then the cancer (if it was still there) would come back. Outpatient surgery turned out to be a pipedream if we wanted things done right.

A few days later, I got a second opinion that completely contradicted his thoughts. And a couple days after that, I had a phone call with a third expert who equivocated between the two. Medicine, it turns out, is art just as often as it is science.

As I struggled with this decision, my mind's eye kept flashing the image of Dr. McLean's large hands holding mine as I asked him question after question.

"How do you get into my chest?" As I spoke, Michael's hand squeezed my thigh, simultaneously comforting me and warning me that the answer was going to be unpleasant.

"Through your sternum," Dr. McLean replied.

I shook my head. "No, I mean, how do you get through my sternum?"

His hands tightened fractionally around mine. "Do you really want to know?"

My head nodded, though my brain was shouting, *ABSOLUTELY FUCKING NOT!*

"With a saw."

I started to cry. Michael's head dropped into his hands.

The room stayed quiet as I wept, letting the emotion wash over and through me. How much more would I need to go through? What else would it take to get back to a life that was familiar, that I understood?

After a puzzling and emotional series of conversations with doctors and Michael and my parents, my thymus was sentenced to a quick death. I sat down to memorialize it for Hair Optional:

MY THYMUS

In general, I'm a fan of my internal organs remaining, well, internal. Our bodies are so complicated and extraordinary that if something is there, it must have a purpose, otherwise it wouldn't be there. Even if medical science does not yet understand what it is.

I know, I've heard the theories about our pinky toes slowly evolving out of the body (I'm sure that women's shoe designers cannot wait for that moment) or the uselessness of, say, the appendix. But then, after years and years of yanking the appendix out of our bodies with nary a second thought, it turns out that it might possibly be an incredibly useful storehouse for good bacteria, which fires into business right when we need it most: during illness.

So when a man in a white coat with his name

embroidered on the left breast with the word *Surgery* underneath tells me that I have an organ with no purpose, I'm going to question him on it.

The thymus is an interesting organ for one that I had never heard of before my surgeon wanted to remove it. It is very flat, lying between the heart and the sternum, with four long arms; two reach up on either side of the neck while the other two reach down alongside the lungs. In some pictures, it almost looks like a butterfly. Vitally important when we are young, it produces T-cells, some of our immune system's best fighters. Its purpose is gradually replaced (or, perhaps, augmented) by bone marrow as we age, resulting in the thymus shrinking and turning almost entirely into fat by the time we are in our seventies, which, according to Western medicine, makes it "useless" after puberty. (If you believe in other schools of thought, the thymus also has a strong hormone regulation purpose and remains active and very important until death.)

Before that fateful day sometime in late adulthood when the immune purpose of the thymus finally and fully self-destructs, it is possible to resuscitate it using herbs and homeopathy, and some studies have shown that adults without a thymus prematurely age. It is not entirely clear how long the thymus remains actively involved in helping the immune system after we reach puberty.

For me, my postchemo PET scan possibly showed "thymic rebound," which means that my thymus was capable of resuscitating itself for at least a few months after having been thoroughly agitated by chemotherapy agents. During those few months, I'd like to think that it was helping out when my bone marrow was too drained to do much. The drug that I was on to help with my immune system during chemo only stimulates bone marrow. Eventually, bone marrow becomes exhausted and stops responding as quickly, or at all, to the stimulation. Which explains why my counts rebounded slower as chemo went on and are expected to take over two years to return to "normal" levels.

My thymus might have already been heading out the door, strangled by a tumor that was, at one point, 12x10x9 cm, and a body that was halfway to seventy. But I don't want you to believe that I let it go quietly into that good night. We checked and double checked, and I had multiple conversations with my angels, demons, friends, and family. Even though my thymus was quiet, I raged, raged against the dying of the light for it.

And now I write this memorial.

I scheduled the surgery for four days after Obama's second inauguration. I figured that the least I could do was let our little family blow off some steam at some fun parties before I had to spend a week in the hospital and then ten weeks recovering at home.

I went to sleep with Dr. McLean and Michael looking down at me, and woke up in recovery with Dr. Levi standing quietly near my bed and Michael dozing with his head near my knees. I had a huge white bandage covering my chest. As I discovered it with my hand, I found tubes dangling out from underneath, and decided to think about that later. Pain medications ran through my veins like a shot of adrenaline, and I tried to tamp down the stimulation and stress, knowing it wouldn't do me any favors.

"How are you feeling?" Dr. Levi asked, taking one of my hands. Her other hand clutched the ever-present iPhone, its headphones dangling around her neck.

I grimaced.

My eyes must have been a little wild, because she checked my morphine drip and hit a few buttons. "You don't want to get to the point where you're feeling pain, but I don't think we need it quite at this level." She grinned. "You'll have to balance the painkilling effects with your response to them."

I croaked something noncommittal.

"The lab has your tumor. In a couple of days, we'll know one way or the other."

"What if it's not gone?" I murmured, trying not to disturb Michael. "What if we did all of this and it's not gone?" Tears started down my cheeks—the opiate-panic kicking into high gear.

"Then we'll deal with it," she replied, "but right now, your job is to recover from surgery."

"I'm scared," I whispered. "I don't want to have cancer anymore."

"Shhhh." Dr. Levi sat down next to me on the bed, cautiously avoiding the tubes. She unplugged her earphones from her phone and laid it by my head. Then she flicked a button, and the quiet tones of a Mozart prelude rose out of my pillow.

"Shhhh, just let the music calm you down. You know how to do this."

I did. I knew how to do this in a hospital bed. Getting present. Staying present. I hiccupped and took a quick breath, then a deeper breath. Then another. I began to match my breathing in and out to the slow beat of the piano. When I woke up again, Michael was asleep on the couch, and Dr. Levi was gone.

Five days later, I was home again, having learned how to clean my new wound that divided my cleavage and how to manage my pain with little residual anxiety, when Dr. Levi knocked on our apartment door. I held the door open, amazed at her presence. Michael stood a few feet behind me, expectantly.

She stood there, in her puffy winter coat, with a grin from ear to ear. "You're fine. You're completely fine. The biopsy showed no evidence of anything."

I burst into tears and hugged her. She hugged me back, and then turned me around and sent me into the arms of my husband. Michael locked his arms around me and held me, gently but as if he would never let go. I nuzzled into his neck and relaxed into his love.

IN APRIL 2013—six months after chemo ended, and two and a half months after my surgery—I found myself on a flight to New York, crouched over the toilet and heaving into the blue chemicals. I had spent the previous night inexplicably throwing up, and by the time the alarm went off at 5 a.m. for my flight, I thought whatever had gone through my system was done. Apparently not.

I'd insisted on making the flight for the visit not only to see my sister, but also because she lives on a farm in the Hudson River Valley. After months of living between my sterile bubble of a high-rise apartment and the sterile bubble of the hospital, I wanted to get dirty, use my muscles, and feel like a human being again. I wanted to feel the ground beneath my feet and dirt under my fingernails. I wanted to remind my psyche that I'm a child of this planet, not a product of sanitized machinery and medical procedures. I wanted to prove that despite the setback of my surgery, I was back on the path to precancer, prechemo strength. And farmwork seemed like the solution.

"What do we need to do?" I asked her as we drove away from the airport.

Corinna glanced at me. "We really need to split wood, actually. We felled a bunch of dying trees, and the logs have been cut into smaller pieces. Now we just need to split and stack them."

"Um, with an axe? How very Paul Bunyan of us." I had no idea how I would even lift an axe, let alone swing it with the force necessary to split a log.

"A friend lent me his splitter, so one of us can use the axe while the other one uses the splitter. And then we can switch."

"Great. I'd like to brush my teeth and have some lunch first, though. I spent the entire flight throwing up."

With the nonchalance of a fellow cancer survivor, she didn't even blink. "Totally reasonable. Let me know if you're going to puke again so I can pull over."

That afternoon found two sisters, one six months out of chemo, the other eight months out of chemo, alternatively wielding an axe and operating a splitter capable of producing what felt like a billion tons of pressure. Like my own cancer experience, Corinna's battle with Hodgkin's lymphoma was tentatively over. But her most recent treatment in Germany was her third chemo protocol, including stem cell replacement therapy, and her fifth medical effort to prevent her ever-dividing cancer cells from blossoming into the illness that had transformed her life seven years earlier. She, too, had been a college rower, and much of her success in life had also been the result of persistence, innate talent, and sheer force of will. So we both crossed our fingers that we were "fine," and got to work bullying our bodies back into health.

The splitter-to-axe production ratio was approximately forty-to-one. Whichever one of us was handling the axe would bring it down on the log, make a small dent, and take a few breaths to recover. Then do it again. We had so little control over the axe that a part of my mind worried one of us would lose a limb. We kept the dog in the house.

When it was my turn at the splitter, I would lean over to the right and take hold of a log. The wood slid through my gloved hands, begging to give me splinters. My biceps, burning and working in concert with the bigger muscles of my back and shoulders, lifted a log into place. The splitter would slowly lower, crushing pulp until it found a seam, and I would hold the pieces apart as the lines gave way. Toss to the left, start over.

And then we would switch. The axe handle, smooth and cool. My triceps and chest contracting to create the force necessary to make even a tiny dent. My ligaments pulling on my bones. My tendons pulling on my muscles. My breath, coming in short bursts, unable to sustain the effort. My mind, remembering some warning, hoping my bones were strong enough to anchor my tendons and ligaments.

But we didn't stop. Adrenals and hearts and muscles be damned! Both of us, frustrated at our bodies' accumulated weakness, kept pushing past our bodies' complaints. Nobody suggested that the gasping breath and inability to swing the axe meant we should stop. Or take a break. Or collapse to the ground and let the dog lick our faces. We knew how stupid we were being, how hard we were pushing ourselves unnecessarily. And the afternoon devolved into the specific hysterics of two kindred spirits who were both facing the same preposterous situation.

After two days of this, my sister and I had split and stacked four cords of wood, and we could barely move. I returned to Chicago ready to drop but confident that the dirt and exercise and comradery and love would force my body to recover.

THE MORNING AFTER my return from the Hudson Valley, I was scheduled to start back to a full day of work for the first time in ten months. On my way out the door, as I leaned over to grab my keys, I found myself grasping the kitchen counter as its cold, smooth surface started floating toward my face. I pushed back, hoping to save my nose from crunching against the counter, before realizing that my face hadn't actually gone anywhere. Despite the wave of nausea flowing through my body, the feeling that I was about to face-plant had been a visual trick.

I was broadsided by a brand-new fear. What was happening to me?

I sat down, had a glass of water, and looked at the cats, who suddenly seemed very interested in why I was pale and a little sweaty. I stumbled to the bathroom, threw up the glass of water, and texted Dr. Levi.

Three hours later, I was in her office. She was on vacation, so I consulted with her nurse practitioner instead. "I'm pretty sure you have benign paroxysmal positional vertigo," he said with a completely straight face.

I burst out laughing, but cut it short as the room began spinning around me. I clutched at my chair and asked him to repeat himself. It turns out that your inner ear contains tiny crystals, and if one gets loose, extreme vertigo can result. And you just have to wait for the crystal to dissolve.

I thought he was joking. My mother had spent my teenage years traumatizing me by becoming a hands-on healer—only wearing white cotton, rearranging all the bedrooms so the head of each bed pointed east or south, and that sort of thing. I'd heard of crystals. They just don't hang out in your ear and make you dizzy.

I was supposed to start work that day, and instead I was sitting in Dr. Levi's office, staring at a wall that wouldn't stay still. Considering that there was nothing to be done about this—I would just have to wait it out—I decided to go to work anyway.

I made it into the law firm's building and carefully navigated to the elevator. To my surprise, I did not fall down when the elevator started to rise. Then I felt my way down the hall to my office and collapsed in the chair with my head between my thighs.

"Is coming back to work really that bad?" Gene had seen me coming and had walked over to say hello.

I informed the floor of my condition. "I have vertigo caused by loose ear crystals."

Gene burst out laughing. "First of all, that doesn't make any sense. Second of all, if you have vertigo, what are you doing here?"

I looked up at him, tears rolling down my face. He closed my door and sat down. I tried to focus on his moving torso and gave up, staring instead at the undulating wall behind him. "What else am I going to do? I've been sick for so long, and I can't keep sitting at home now that I'm mostly better. Plus, you and the firm have been great. I owe you so much."

"What? Is that seriously why you're here? You can't even see straight, let alone read or write!"

"Sometimes it's not so bad," I sniffled.

"I'm going to walk you downstairs and hail you a cab. Please don't come back until you can walk without holding on to the walls."

Three days later, I was sitting in front of Dr. Levi, who was just back from London. She was staring at me with an incredulous look on her face. "Ear crystals?"

"Hey, I'm just relaying information here."

She shook her head as she typed out a prescription. "I'm going to give you something to see if this is actually vertigo. If it isn't better in two days, let me know."

"Okay, but what do I have?"

"I don't know. My best guess is that you caught a bug of some sort a couple of weeks ago, and you're just taking a long time to clear it. Don't forget, I beat the shit out of your bone marrow last year."

I went home, swallowed her solution, and went to bed. In

the morning, the walls still wobbled, but I went to work anyway. This time, I stayed the whole day and came home with an assignment that I could barely read. Michael put me to bed with bone broth, a cat, and a kiss. When I woke up the following morning, the room didn't lurch to one side. Finally.

The next day was a full one. I had breakfast with a friend, worked the entire day, dealt with household finances, went for a walk, cuddled the cats, chatted with my sister on the phone, and had a lovely dinner with Michael. Then I fell into bed, utterly shattered.

At work the following morning, Gene walked into my office, closed the door behind him, and sat down. "We need to talk." He looked and sounded serious, which was unusual for him, so I ignored it.

"About the fact that you're not moving around anymore?" I grinned. "Because that's totally worth talking about."

He didn't smile. "Yes and no, you crazy person."

Uh-oh, this sounds serious. I turned away from my computer. "What's up?"

"You're exhausted." It wasn't a question.

I looked at him quizzically. "True, but that's to be expected. Dr. Levi said I'm going to be tired for at least two years postchemo. That doesn't mean I should just stay in bed until I'm better."

"Nobody's suggesting that you just stay in bed until you're fully recovered, especially if it takes that long. But what are you doing here?" He gestured around my barren Big Law office.

Confused, and a little hurt that he wasn't recognizing the massive effort it took just to be sitting in my office, I responded sharply, "What do you mean? This is my job."

His eyes softened. "Lydia, this is me. I sat with you during chemo. I brought you food and games and laughter when you felt good. I brought you food and movies when you were recovering from surgery. I even brought you work when you insisted on it. We are friends. *What are you doing here?*"

The air went out of me, and I collapsed in on myself. I swung my seat back to my computer and logged on to my health insurance account. Then I pushed a few buttons and turned the monitor so he could see what I was doing. "This is how much my care has cost this law firm since I was diagnosed last June." The number flashing across the top of the screen was unfathomable: $757,993.46.

"I know, some percentage of this was negotiated away, and another percentage just disappeared into the morass of our broken health care system. But this firm has given me three-quarters of a million dollars' worth of health care, let alone my salary and short-term disability and long-term disability, and asked me for *nothing* in return. I owe them." I stared at him, willing him to understand. For some reason, it was vitally important that he comprehend this need for me to be working.

"Yeah, you mentioned that before. And I still think you're putting too much pressure on yourself. You don't owe us anything. That's why we have insurance. That's why there is more than one person here who is capable of doing your job. Sometimes people get sick, and the fact that we could help was something that gave the partners pride. They *wanted* to help you. Nobody is expecting anything out of you. Give them some credit."

I tried a different tack. "If I don't do this, what do I do? I spent three years and two hundred fifty thousand dollars gathering all these ridiculous degrees." I waved my arm in the direction of my wall of certificates and diplomas. "And I'm not about to let that go to waste just because I had cancer for a few months."

"And surgery. Don't forget your surgery."

My fingers absently rubbed my scar—my mark of Cain—through my shirt, feeling the bumps under my skin where wires were holding my sternum together. "Oh, don't worry, I don't ever forget my damn surgery. I'm never going to be able to wear a V-neck again."

Sympathy oozed from Gene. He tried again. "How do I put it? You . . ." He paused. "You hate it here."

I smiled. "I don't hate it here. I'm overwhelmed by the idea of working twelve-to-fourteen-hour days again. God knows I don't have the patience to Lean In anymore. But how am I ever going to recover if I don't try to get back to my life?"

He looked a little stunned. "Jumping into the deep end seems like a dramatic way to get back to your life."

"What else would you suggest?" I kept smiling and talking before he had a chance to answer. "I have friends like you to keep me entertained and join me for pasta at lunch once a week. I feel like that is a solid starting point toward keeping me sane." I was still reaching toward my old familiar life, and frustrated that people kept questioning me on it. The fact that it was harder than I had expected was something I tried to ignore. I was searching for comfortable, but every time I thought I would find it—including this time, at work—it would shift out of reach once again. This was very annoying.

Gene fixed me with his stare. "Be serious."

I stopped smiling. "I am being serious. I need to be doing

something to remind my sluggish brain and my wasted body that I'm a useful member of humanity. I know how to do this, and I have no energy to find something else that may be less taxing. Let me give this place a year. Just a year. Then, if I'm still battling reality, you can come back and yell at me again."

He contemplated my offer. "What does Michael think about all this?"

"He thinks I'm being ridiculous too. But he understands my need to feel useful."

Gene sighed, stood up, and started poking at his phone. "I'm putting a note in my calendar for one year from today: *Yell at Lydia*. He walked to the door and paused. "Lunch? It's pasta day!"

MY COMPLEX RELATIONSHIP with my job was further complicated—mentally, emotionally, and at times, practically—by my continuing tango with my doctors, the hospital, and my health. A month after I went back to work, the day after a follow-up CT scan, I got an overly cheerful text message from Dr. Levi sharing that I still didn't have cancer.

I was delighted that I remained out of the grasp of medicine. But the news didn't bring me the solace that I thought it would. Instead, it rang hollow as a speed limit sign on an empty, straight road in the desert. Because a part of me had been hoping that my CT scan wouldn't be clean, that I would have to go in for a full month to do a stem-cell replacement.

Of course, this was insane. This stem-cell treatment is one round of chemotherapy so powerful that it basically kills your entire immune system, and then you're brought back to health through an infusion of either your own or someone else's stem cells. I've witnessed this treatment with my sister, and the fact that a small part of my brain actively wished for it should have had me begging for a lobotomy.

So here's my dirty secret: from the first minute that I went back to work, all I wanted was to go back to the hospital. Despite the fact that being sick is horrible and undergoing chemo is even worse, the hospital itself felt secure to me. In all my adult life, it was the only place I had ever felt truly comfortable. I knew exactly why I was there and what I was supposed to do while there. I was a control freak with nothing to control, so I could finally rest.

In the hospital, there were no questions. There was no living in the future, because it was impossible to even joke about plans posttreatment, let alone make them. There was no living in the past, because other than family and friends, no form of my past life existed. I lived, diligently and exhaustedly and often hilariously, fully in the present. And for this gift, I loved that building with my entire being. I loved the nurses and techs and other staff. I loved my view of the lake and the hard-plastic mattress and raising my head with the touch of a button. I loved the plain and simple fact that I had nothing in my day-to-day life to question.

But now, I had a blank slate. Instead of being mentally present with no choices, I was mentally present with infinite choices, and the burden of those choices was crushing me. Graduating from patient to survivor ripped my fragile sense of calm from my desperate fingers.

Two months passed. Day after day, I sat at work, staring

at my wall where I had hung a poster of my favorite beach. I had been doing good work, staying appropriate hours, cracking jokes when it seemed like the right moment. My fatigue pulled at me, though. I wanted to crawl into the picture and go for a quiet walk on that beautiful, soft sand. I wanted to let the blue of the sky and the green of the ocean envelop my body. Floating on the salt water would give me the space I needed to listen to my body and quiet my mind, to figure out what I wanted to do.

My brain was different now. I didn't have the patience for complex problems, although I had discovered unlimited patience for more menial data management work. I could do the hard work, but where my brain used to slide effortlessly through it, staying focused was now a perpetual battle.

With a sigh, feeling like an imposter in my mind, I turned to my computer and pulled up a draft brief that was due in a few days. This document was for one of the very few women partners in the group, someone I had made an effort to work with before I got sick and had hoped to avoid the minute I came back. We were the same age, but my varied career choices put me well behind her in the firm hierarchy. Although she tried to mentor me, something about our pairing didn't quite work. She also had a bad habit of micromanaging me as though I were a first-grader. Before I got sick, I saw this as a challenge. I could absolutely play the game of corporate law and office rat race. Afterward, I just didn't care.

To me, this partner's need for control was as exhausting as wearing the high heels that now collected dust in my closet. With the retirement of my heels had gone makeup and tailored outfits. My spiky pixie cut negated any need for effort with my hair. My work uniform now consisted of trousers made of stretchy material, flats, sweaters, and a designer scarf—comfort with just enough style to avoid being told, by one of the senior women partners whose job it was to make sure the women associates don't embarrass themselves, that women need to look a certain way. Given what some of the men wore every day, I know for a fact that there was no senior gentleman who had a similar job description.

Although I never missed a deadline or a meeting, I passive-aggressively refused to be micromanaged. I dropped by the partner's office every now and again to say hi and check in; but otherwise, I stared at my beach or went to therapy appointments. When I was unceremoniously dumped from her team, I took myself out to dinner to celebrate.

The most fun I had upon my return to work involved a legal brawl between a bankrupt client and one of its unions. I was working for a different partner then, one who informed me at the beginning of our relationship that he didn't give a shit where I worked or when I worked or how I worked, as long as I did a good job and completed assignments when he needed them. He was the perfect boss for my new state of mind.

The legal problem involved contract interpretation. I have never been a tremendous fan of unions in their modern incarnation, and this particular one was demanding the client pay more than the contract required for its pension. Because of arbitration and all the rest, case law in state court said the union was entitled to the inflated pension, despite the words in the contract. The trick was to draft a brief that pointed the federal bankruptcy judge back to the words of the contract and, essentially, to ignore the ruling of the state court.

I loved it. All of my history of managing large institutions in government fed into solving this particular problem. The tension was subtle and complex: Federal judges hate being told what to do by state judges. State judges hate the superiority of federal judges. Bankruptcy judges, a subset of the federal system, love thumbing their nose at all of them. And playing various players off of each other was my specialty.

In any legal problem or dispute, Law 101 commands that you always go back to the words of the law, contract, or regulation. If the language is unclear, only then do you go to other sources—legislative history, case law, historic practices—for help interpreting it. For case law, there's a strict hierarchy of precedence, and it's all dependent on whether a judge is interpreting a federal law issue or a state law issue. Even though bankruptcy judges are in the federal system, if they're interpreting a state law issue, they have to look to state case law for help in interpreting it. That is, unless there is a federal bankruptcy opinion on the exact same issue, in which case the judge is held to that—but only if it's an opinion written by a court that actually has authority over that particular judge.

It's complicated, but it's not rocket science. This particular issue was complicated in a way that I loved. It was intellectual gamesmanship.

But then I thought about the case beyond the legal problem displayed on my computer screen. Our client was doing much better financially than the twelve members of this tiny union who simply wanted a little help with their pension fund. My fees to draft the brief and the partner's fees to review the brief totaled more than what the union wanted. A part of me understood the fight: if the client settled here, then others would come to the company with their hands out. Another part of me just wanted to donate my fees to the union and solve the problem for these truck drivers who earned less than I did while I was on disability.

Legally, it was cut and dried. But ethically, morally? Not so simple. And this dilemma grated on me much more loudly than it had before I got sick.

ONE OF THE FEW true delights during my days back at work involved walking to and from my office. Chicago is so beautiful in the summer, and the forty-five-minute walk each direction nurtured me in ways that nothing else could.

On my walk home one day, I tripped over the curb and a friendly stranger seized my arm before a passing cab creamed me.

I smiled at him and spoke automatically. "Thank you so much!" The empathy of a fellow human shone in his kind eyes. Yet a bizarre set of emotions rose up in me. Not gratitude. Not relief. Not the calm as a surge of adrenaline quiets. Instead, I felt disappointment and despair.

I stopped and stood back against the brick wall of some office building, letting the foot traffic stream by me as I wrestled with these emotions. Feelings of confusion had been building inside me for months, overflowing at strange moments as I tried to integrate back into work. They had shown themselves previously in my traitorous distress every time Dr. Levi gave me more good news. In that moment of being saved from a traumatic accident, a new emotion layered on top: fear. The diabolical voice in the back of my mind—the one that wanted to go back to the hospital, that wanted to stop living this strange life of a postcancer patient—was getting louder. I was so desperate to go back to the hospital, I actually was beginning to welcome the idea of getting hit by a car.

It didn't make sense. Of course I didn't want cancer again. But I wanted anything that would put me back into the place where my control freak had no role—where my mind stayed quiet, I felt calm, and my body could be strong or weak or skinny or fat, and such concerns didn't matter because healing was paramount.

Although there is much to celebrate when once faces down an existential threat—when the sum total of a year's accomplishments are *staying alive* and *staying married*—at the time, those accomplishments felt empty. They paled in comparison to my life before. Now, *alive* meant "barely functioning," and *married* meant "happy but still very fragile." I knew what my life had looked like before everything had fallen apart—health, strength, honeymoon love—and there was no part of my life as a survivor that looked the same as it once had. At least in the hospital, I had an excuse for feeling like an imposter in my own body and life.

Bottom line: I couldn't continue to be defined by my health status. I desperately needed an external definition that meant I'd achieved something beyond survival.

By the way, my client won that contract interpretation case against the union.

FERTILITY

DURING THE YEAR after chemo, my desperation to return to the hospital was in fact a deep desire to return to living in the present—I understand this now. In my hospital bed, the present was all I could count on, so I lived moment by moment. But out in the real world, I had no idea how to do that. I had no reference point other than the way I had always lived my life: as a control freak.

At work, it became depressingly clear that I was failing to control how my brain now functioned. So instead, I desperately tried to control my body. Everything was different: hair, muscles, hormones. Everything. I still had no desire to have a baby, but I wanted my body to get back to my version of normal. Getting my period back on track at age thirty-four seemed like an obvious place to start.

Thirteen months after my previous period visited me in a haze of bony pain and opiates, I bled again. Sort of. This seemed like such an amazing piece of news that instead of simply being grateful for it, I immediately took myself off to a gynecologist who had come highly recommended for being kind to postchemo patients. I learned, not for the first time in my life, that not all reputations are deserved.

I told this doctor multiple times during my visit that I didn't want children at the moment, if ever. I just wanted to know what was going on with my hormones. Who knows what she heard, but it wasn't what I said. Or maybe some doctors only target the results and not the causes. Or maybe she was having a bad day. Or maybe she is just truly terrible at her job. Whatever the reason, I got caught in the middle.

A few weeks after I saw her and gave multiple vials of blood for multiple tests, the gynecologist called me with the results. I was standing in line at Whole Foods with my friend Ynez, buying food for a dinner party due to start in my apartment approximately five minutes later.

"So, one of the numbers is too high," the doctor intoned, "and something else is too low, and blah blah blah postmenopausal blah blah blah . . ."

Ynez, watching my face go white at the word *postmenopausal*, turned around and grabbed the first bottle of wine she saw, adding it to the basket alongside the lettuce and quinoa.

". . . blah blah blah we can speak to the fertility people at the hospital but something else on your results makes me think egg harvesting won't work and . . . Remind me of your timeline for wanting children?"

I handed my credit card to the cashier. "At the moment, never. But not for another year at least. I still haven't hit my one-year anniversary from finishing chemo."

"Oh, right. Well, even so, you might want to think about egg donors." Was she listening to anything coming out of my mouth?

"Could any of this be related to the fact that I'm still clearing everything out of my system?" I asked as we exited the store.

"Possibly," she replied, "but I'm fairly convinced that little period you had was just a blip."

"Have you ever seen anything like this before with your postchemo patients?" I turned to Ynez in the evening light and widened my eyes, not sure exactly what I was telling her, but knowing something was wrong with either me or the doctor on the other end of the line. "Because both my oncologist and my acupuncturist told me it takes a lot of energy to build a full uterine lining, so even though it was really only five days of spotting, they're fairly sure that I actually cycled. You disagree?"

Ynez returned my look, and as we walked the few blocks to my apartment, concern filled her eyes.

"Every patient is different, but right now your tests are telling me that you are postmenopausal." The doctor's voice smacked of efficiency but lacked any kind of emotion.

I suddenly realized that if I was going to get through life postchemo, people like this were entirely useless to me. "Well, um, thanks, I guess. Could you please send me the test results?" This woman knew barely anything about me and had the bedside manner of the Grinch. I had no idea if her medical diagnosis was accurate, but to my mind, the strength of her convictions after only one blood test and no physical exam made her entirely unqualified.

"I'll put them in the mail."

That was it. No *I'm sorry to have to tell you this,* no *maybe we should get an ultrasound*, no *maybe we should wait another few months to take another test*.

Ynez, my beautiful, creative friend, had been through her own experience with hormone tests and needles and ultrasounds because she was single at age thirty-five and didn't know what else to do amid the media onslaught about how she was losing her chance to have a child.

"What are your actual numbers?" she asked.

"I have no idea."

"How remarkably irresponsible."

The street lost its color. Ynez took my hand as we walked. I couldn't find . . . the right . . . spot . . . to put . . . my . . . feet. I tripped over a crack in the sidewalk. Everyone was walking faster than normal. When we ran into another friend in the lobby of my building, she and Ynez spoke at hyperspeed while I leaned against the back of the elevator. Then we were inside my apartment, and Ynez was handing me a glass of wine and encouraging me to take large gulps. Michael got home, took me into the bedroom, and held me while I wept. More friends showed. I took a deep breath and waited a minute for time to right itself, went out to our living room, said hello, gave hugs, poured more wine, and sat down. Then I exploded.

"You guys are all really close friends so you might as well know that my new gynecologist called me this evening to inform me, after one blood test, that I'm probably infertile and should find an egg donor."

The men lifted their drinks to their mouths and sat back in their chairs. The women sat up straighter, their righteous indignation flowing across the table.

"One blood test?" said one.

"Did she recommend an ultrasound?" said another.

"Do you want the name of my gynecologist? Yours sounds like a nightmare," said a third.

"Oh, sweetie," said Ynez.

"Have you spoken to Dr. Levi?" asked Elizabeth.

Their love and unwillingness to accept some doctor's conclusion was so bolstering to me that I immediately calmed down. *There is no part of my life that isn't working if I have these friends at my dinner table*, I thought.

One of my closest friends, who was five months pregnant after a year of trying, was quiet and looked stricken. I reached out and clasped her hand in mine. "Stop it. Whatever is going through your head right now, *stop* it. I'm thrilled for you. This is my problem, and it doesn't make me any less happy for you or mad at you or anything. So knock it off."

She grimaced.

I poured another glass of wine.

I woke up that night baking in my own personal radiator, swimming in a puddle of sweat. This hot flash was worse than normal, which I had expected given the amount of wine I had consumed. I got out of bed quietly and started moving through my night sweat routine while waiting for my body heat to dissipate. Pull back the comforter to give it air. Remove the soaked towel from under my body. Wrench a new T-shirt from the pile on my dresser. Change shirts. Take a deep breath. And another.

I soaked a washcloth in cold water and started wiping down the back of my neck. Within seconds, the washcloth was as hot as my skin.

A few months previously, Michael and I were at an outdoor concert, his arms wrapped around me to keep me warm.

Suddenly, I pulled out of his arms, unzipped my jacket, and unbuttoned my sweater. He grinned, by that time used to my fluctuating hormones, and asked, "Is that what it's like every time? You feel like you just peed yourself." Yes, that's what it was like. At least five times a day. Since chemo began.

That night in my bedroom, as I stared at myself in the mirror for ages, sweat mingled with the tears dripping down my face. I wondered if my body would ever get back to normal, and I found myself begging it, willing it to do so. Then, a few minutes after I had gotten out of bed, I flipped my pillow over and crawled under the damp comforter, shaking a little from the cold sweat drying on my body.

It took me three days to recover from my dinner party hangover. Cancer cells love alcohol, which is pure sugar, so I'd stopped drinking during chemo and never really got back into the habit. The three glasses of wine that night simply annihilated my system. My brain couldn't write or form complex thoughts until the following week, when I called the onco-fertility specialist whom I had first met while panicked in the hospital three days after someone in the ER told me I had cancer.

"Gah! Blood tests! Infertile! Gynecologist wants me to get an egg donor!"

"Hi, Lydia. Um, what?"

I explained what had happened.

"Please send me your labs," she said, "and I'll be happy to meet with you and Michael tomorrow. In the meantime, please remember that the only thing these labs are is a baseline."

"What do you mean?"

"Now we know where you were as of August 3, 2013, thirteen

months after starting chemo. These tests don't mean you are infertile. They just mean your body is still recovering from chemo, which you already knew. Okay?"

I took a deep breath. "Okay."

For the next thirty-six hours, a new mantra ran through my head: *just a baseline . . . just a baseline . . .*

Michael and I met the specialist the following day at the tea shop in the hospital lobby. She gave us each a hug before we sat down in a private corner. When she started talking, I could almost see her words creating a shape like a small animal, crouching and cowering on the table. The creature was wondering if I would gather it up in my arms and accept it, or drop-kick it through the plate-glass window in front of me.

As I found out then, testing AMH (anti-Müllerian hormone), which gynecologists love because it reports on ovarian reserves, is a useless measure for women immediately post-chemo. It measures the hormone released by eggs that are in the middle stage of development—not those about to pop and, most important for me, not the little ones that have yet to emerge. Women whose cycle has never been interrupted for any reason usually have three or four of these mid-stage eggs on the back burner, so the test tends to start high at puberty and generally decreases until it hits zero at menopause. Therefore, all the gynecologist's test told me was that my ovaries, as of the test date, had not yet restarted. Because of my continuing hot flashes, this was information I already knew.

The other test we discussed was on FSH (follicle-stimulating hormone), which in my case was off-the-charts high. This one measures how loudly the pituitary gland is shouting at the ovaries, telling them to activate estrogen in order to coax a mid-stage egg into final development so it can be released for the monthly cycle. Once the pituitary gland senses estrogen, it shuts FSH down—but if no estrogen is present, then it just keeps sending FSH. So, once again, the tests simply showed that my ovaries were not yet responding.

"So what does all of this mean?" I asked, not sure if I wanted to hear the answer.

The specialist shook her head. "Absolutely nothing."

"Um, it sounds like it means a lot."

"What these tests say is that you are postchemo, which we already knew."

I turned that one over in my head for a minute. There had to be something important she wasn't telling me. "When do I stop being postchemo?"

"When your body is ready."

I'd had this conversation before. With Dr. Levi. With Ruth. With Michael. With Corinna. With my acupuncturist. With my personal trainer. With my yoga teacher. With about nine thousand people. I was certifiably sick of having this conversation.

I glared at the specialist.

She relented, with a small, indulgent smile. "Okay. It takes women anywhere from six to eighteen months before their hormones reset into their 'new normal.' So if you insist on knowing when you are done with this aspect of chemo, it will be anytime from four months ago until April 2015."

My face locked into stubborn mode. "This is not helpful information."

"Well, I can't give you more than that." The corner of her

mouth twitched into an even bigger smile as she watched me get more stubborn. Her eyes softened. "Why did you go to the gynecologist in the first place?" she quietly asked.

"I wanted to know what was going on."

"Why? Do you want a child right now?"

The question snapped me out of my frown, and I laughed. "Good lord, no!" I could barely walk after the damage that chemo did to my knee ligaments and tendons. I was barely functioning at the office. Every time I had a hot flash, I started hyperventilating about whether I had cancer again. But I was almost thirty-five years old, and even without chemo, my biological alarm clock was already ringing. Which was really weird because I still didn't want to have kids.

She smiled. "So what you're telling me is that you went to the gynecologist because you're a control freak and a glutton for punishment."

Shit.

I closed my mouth, which had dropped open, and cradled my head in my hands. "If it makes any difference," I mumbled to her via my knees, "I'm trying to be less of a control freak."

Michael laughed. "To her credit, she really is."

I looked at him and smiled, grateful for the support.

The specialist grinned and turned to me. "Well, you're not doing a very good job of it, at least on this count." She gave me two options: Go and get this blood test every month, and keep myself in a constant state of panic about whether my ovaries were recovering. Or stop worrying about it, and when Michael and I actually decide we want a child, then try to have a child. "Then, if it doesn't work, come back to me. We're doing all kinds of astounding research into postchemo fertility, and we'll be able to help."

Michael responded first: "I vote for option two."

She laughed. I chuckled weakly.

We sat for another few moments as I turned the conversation over in my head, looking for more information and knowing that it wasn't there. Then I, too, cast my vote for option two.

OUR BODIES DON'T LIE. Only our minds lie. The body sends off a twinge, and the mind's job is to interpret it. Whatever the mind produces—from *Just a scratch* to *Holy shit, my thumb just fell off!*—is an interpretation of the body's honest signal. This goes beyond potential crisis moments such as whether a paper cut needs stitches. This goes to the crap that our mind does to our body all the time. Feeding it junk food and sugar and unhealthy meat and not enough clean water. Smoking. Breathing exhaust fumes and industrial chemicals. Exercising too hard. Exercising too little. Not eating enough veggies. Swallowing too many medications we don't need. Living a life of stress. Living in toxic relationships. Shying away from abundance and love.

Inside all of this mind garbage, our poor body is not just trying to survive but constantly working to thrive, to be healthy and whole. The body constantly cleans out toxins and floods of adrenaline, tries to process too much sugar, and does it all with not enough actual nutrition and not enough water, so we hold weight as our body literally builds a bubble of protection from the onslaught.

Sometimes, however, the body-mind syncs up and truly

magical stuff happens. You finally say that thing you've been meaning to say, and your sore throat goes away. You finally ask for, and receive, support for something, and your lower back pain goes away. You finally grieve a loss and forgive yourself for something, and your shoulders lighten. You learn to meditate, and your chronic migraines ease off.

In my case, I decided to stop worrying about my hormones, and two days later my hot flashes stopped, and four days later my period emphatically reappeared. I bled for a full cycle once every fourteen to eighteen days for the better part of six months. I decided to start living in the present, and my body rewarded me. Huh. How about that?

SOMETHING ELSE HAPPENED during that conversation in the quiet corner of the hospital lobby. This lovely woman informed me that she had been poking through the Internet in some previous moment and had found my blog post ranting about the fertility process at the hospital, and how it was not very user-friendly for cancer patients. She had looked into what I had written and, as a result, encouraged the hospital to make some changes.

Because of something I had done, the enormous machine of hospital-land became a little friendlier to women who were simultaneously frightened for their lives and for their quality of life. I had created meaningful change without even knowing it.

I held on to this piece of information in the back of my head from that day forward. As I returned to my job, writing and speaking words on behalf of clients who, for the most part, were prioritizing human greed over humanity, I felt that perhaps I had a different path ahead of me. For the first time, the potential of my future felt more nurturing and full of potential than my past.

AS MY PERIOD began to show up more regularly, my weight exploded. The twenty pounds I had needed to gain since chemo ended were quickly overtaken by another fifteen. Dr. Levi was thrilled: "Your hormone system is restarting!" I was not.

Someone would ask how I was doing, and it would take all of my willpower not to burst into tears. I jokingly told friends that I felt like I was dating my own body. The part I didn't share was that I didn't like my new partner. It was lazy, fat, and weak. My body craved long walks on the beach and gentle massages. Meanwhile, my brain craved a long run followed by yoga.

My body was just different now. I had played two varsity sports in high school and one in college. As an adult, I went for six-mile runs on a whim and practiced yoga regularly. This gave me a slender, strong body and days that started with an endorphin rush and the focus that came with it. In the past, I had built confidence in my body and my physical strength, which translated to emotional strength and confidence in my actions. That body was no longer present. I was an athlete trapped in an unathletic body, and it gnawed at me like a tapeworm. I couldn't even acknowledge the feminine beauty that fertility had brought back to my body—the soft curves, the signs of being nourished and able to carry life, of being alive.

"Your porn showed up today!" Michael would yell as he tossed me the Athleta catalog. This had become a joke between us. For an athlete recovering from chemo, this catalog bordered on an unhealthy fixation. I would hungrily flip the pages, stopping at six-pack abs, defined quads, and a particularly ridiculous version of a forearm stand. He would watch, concerned, until I would toss the catalog into the recycling bin, turn to him with a smile, and say, "Someday."

His response was invariably a kiss to the cheek. "Whenever you're ready."

I started doing what I had always done when my body and I were out of sync: I overruled it. In response to my fifteen pounds of "extra" flesh, I started running again. And then immediately stopped because I couldn't breathe.

This was a temporary problem. After doing a little research, I bought a heart rate monitor and figured out that my heart rate simply wouldn't go above 120. My heart wasn't capable of delivering oxygen to my muscles at the rate that I needed it. With heart rate monitor in hand, I started doing intervals on the treadmill. After a month, it crept up to 130. Another month got me to 140. Another month—160. I would tumble into the shower and then into bed after every workout, mentally and physically beat.

Then new problems began when I realized it would take me up to ten minutes to come down from 160. Intervals, by necessity, had to get shorter as the breaks got longer. Furious, I increased my time on the treadmill and bullied my body into believing it didn't need the amount of oxygen that it actually did. I lost weight, but the workout never gave me the burst of energy I used to enjoy. Instead, I was dog-tired.

And it wasn't just the cardio. I was back in the gym with

weights, finding more proof that my wasted body couldn't do what it once could, and perpetually weeping as a result. Instead of being proud that my face was red from exertion instead of pale green (before diagnosis) or white (right after chemo), I was frustrated that it was round instead of defined. Instead of congratulating myself on moving from no weights for a bicep curl to three-pound weights and then, miraculously, five-pound weights, I was frustrated that the weights weren't ten or fifteen pounds.

My meditation practice, so important to me during chemo, had fallen by the wayside. My ability to stay grounded in the present and take pride in what was true, instead of building a story around what should or could exist, fell along with it. For whatever reason, the importance and urgency I felt around getting my body "back to normal" trumped any mental or spiritual health benefit of quieting my mind. I couldn't hold both concepts together at the same time. Every time I tried, my enduring exhaustion got in the way. So I went with what had been familiar for my thirty-plus years instead of what had been comfortable in recent months: body first, mind and spirit later.

MAY 1, 2014. My one-year deadline to quit my job passed, and I hoped that Michael wouldn't say anything. He looked at me, but kept quiet. Gene didn't keep his appointment either. I sat at my computer, obsessively listening to "Defying Gravity" from the *Wicked* soundtrack, and wept.

My muscles burned from my most recent workout; my heart beat frantically inside my chest. Over the weekend, at an art festival, I had purchased a photograph of a young black girl wearing a white dress, standing on a white porcelain sink surrounded by white tile and a huge mirror in what appeared to be a public bathroom—her arms outstretched, her face reflected in the mirror, a combination of mischief and awe and excitement and a little fear.

I loved her from the minute I saw her out of the corner of my eye as I walked by her uncle's photography booth. I asked him what the expression on her face was about. A consummate artist, he responded, "What do you see?"

In reality, she was breaking the rules—her mother had just told her not to climb onto the sink. But what I saw was her joy at the possibilities in front of her outweighing her nervousness about the uncertainty over those possibilities. Michael had laughed in delight while watching me fall in love with the picture. He immediately dubbed her *your girl*, as in "Are you taking your girl to work with you?"

"Obviously," I responded, squeezing his hand.

I was getting there. I was getting back to "normal." My body was getting "stronger." My work was getting easier to palate. And despite this progress, I had never been more uncomfortable.

I had done everything I was "supposed" to do. I had submitted to the surgery. I had gone back to work. I had seen my therapist. I had registered for the obligatory *I'm healthy!* foot race. I had been working my body despite it begging me to stop.

Unlike in my previous life, "healthy" felt entirely wrong. My lungs battled for air. At work, the walls felt close and brutally unfriendly, my various certificates and degrees and mental achievements mocking me.

Tears rolled down my cheek as I searched my photograph for answers. Why wasn't I enraptured by the possibilities, like my little girl? Why wasn't I happy or focused or strong? I had followed all the instructions. I had gone back to work. I had gone back to the gym. My sense of betrayal started creeping in around the edges as I stared at her quiet defiance, her serene attitude toward the uncertainty of life. I could almost see her eyes as a mirror staring back at me, encouraging me to climb onto the sink with her, stretch my arms out, and fly with joy toward the future—leaving my battered plan to return to "health" on the white bathroom floor.

HEART

STARTING SOON AFTER the surgery to remove my thymus and what remained of my dead tumor, my dreams shifted. I've always had magnificent flying dreams, but these were different.

In these dreams, I was the recipient of the infamous "death by a thousand cuts" torture scenario. I found myself at a cocktail party, tied down to the dining room table amid a haze of alcohol and perfume, surrounded by guests sipping glasses of prosecco and cabernet and casually nicking my prone body while discussing whatever intrigued them.

I was whipped or otherwise beaten as part of a ritualized group torture session. Five people, including myself, would be sitting comfortably in a plush, darkened room. Another small group would whip or beat us up with the efficiency and emotion of robots. We would not complain—quite the opposite, we would be chatting amongst ourselves as the atrocities were performed on our bodies. Sometimes I would be observing, leaning up against the wall, but mostly I was methodically brutalized.

A group of men would focus on me as one would focus on

an unfinished and undesired project, remove my clothing, and systematically rape me. Multiple times.

I describe these dreams with the clinical emotion that I felt while having them. Although the scenes were extremely violent, I had the emotional bandwidth of a detached observer both during and after the dream. I never felt fear or pain, disgust or outrage. I simply noticed that this extraordinary violence was meted out as if perfectly normal.

I tend not to think of myself as a sociopath, yet I was so apathetic to the violence in these dreams that I began to wonder about my emotional stability.

Ruth and I were sitting in her office, and I'd just finished describing my most recent torture, still very present in my mind. "In Jungian dream interpretation," she commented, "all of these are medical dreams."

I looked up at her, hope warming my chest. "So I'm not a sociopath?"

She grinned. "No, Lydia, you're not a sociopath."

According to this way of looking at things, what we sometimes choose to do to our body through the invasiveness of Western medicine requires our psyche to detach from our physical self. In some cases, as with chemotherapy and sternum-cracking, the "medicine" is so violent that our body simply does not understand why our mind is not fighting against the procedure. Our physical side feels cut off and abandoned by the part of us—the rational mind—designed to protect us from physical harm.

Dreams like these, which feature emotional detachment coupled with violence, were my body's way of trying to process what I had chosen to do to it. Little did I know, my body was about to be forced to sort out another medical intrusion.

AFTER DR. MCLEAN sawed my sternum in half to pull out my thymus, he wrapped the flat, wide bone with wire to keep it in place while the bone knitted back together. This procedure involved threading wire around the sternum in a loop; bringing the two ends together; twisting them off; and burying them back into my sternum so they wouldn't poke up through my skin and cause lacerations, infections, and pain. Generally, the twisted-off nubbin is not that big of a deal. However, because I was emaciated from chemo, the little nubbins stuck up like mosquito bites. And because I was compulsive about the fact that I had just had major surgery, and therefore touched these little nubbins all the time, I had six little bruises marching down the center of my chest, like green buttons next to the red zipper of my scar.

Dr. McLean told me that if I stopped touching them, they would stop hurting. He also told me that if I gained weight, they would become less obvious and more cushioned with fat, solving the problems of both appearance and pain. So I sat on my hands and waited. And waited. And waited.

When my hormones restarted and my weight exploded, part of the problem did resolve. But there was one nubbin, up near my collarbone, that refused to be buried in fat and kept hurting. Every time I wore a necklace, it would activate. Every time I wore a particular workout top, it would trigger. Every time I turned my head too far to the right, it would push back. And every time I would flinch as it made itself known, my mind and spirit would plummet in a downward spiral of internal haranguing: *I was fine before the surgery so I didn't really need the surgery except to tell me that I was fine before the surgery and now I have a* HUGE FUCKING SCAR *ripping my chest in half with a fucking wire nubbin under my skin that shoots off a throbbing pain every time I wear a necklace to try to cover up the* HUGE FUCKING SCAR *ripping my chest in half.*

Inspiring, it was not.

Partially because of the physical pain, but mostly because of the emotional pain, I went back to Dr. McLean eighteen months after the surgery and told him the stupid nubbin had to go. While I was at it, I also reached out to a plastic surgeon and told him that the red, chelated scar dividing my chest also had to go.

This surgery happened on July 15, 2014, two years after diagnosis and fourteen months after I returned to work. I came out of it with no sternal wires and a thin, white, flat, beautiful scar. And something else was new: a fairly intense shortness of breath, especially when I leaned over with my head below my heart. The "weird breathing thing," as I called it, lasted about a week—solved through a combination of Advil and acupuncture. Then it came back with a vengeance two weeks later.

It was bad enough that when I texted Dr. Levi about it, on August 11, she asked me to come in that afternoon for a chest X-ray. Because extreme shortness of breath was one of my symptoms when I was first diagnosed—resulting from the tumor pushing on my heart, lungs, and veins—she wanted to see what was going on.

For so long, part of me wanted nothing more than to go back to the hospital, where I was forced out of uncertainty and into the present. Now I realized once and for all that my wish was beyond stupid.

That afternoon, I met Michael at Dr. Levi's office, got a chest X-ray and a blood draw, and waited for the news: the X-ray was clear, and my blood work remained excellent. We had no idea why the shortness of breath had returned, but as long as it didn't have anything to do with cancer and Advil could fix it, I didn't particularly care. As we left, Dr. Levi reminded me that I was also due for my semiannual cancer-maintenance CT scan.

Over the course of the week, the breathing problems eased a bit. They were not the focus of my attention when I went into the hospital on the morning of August 15 for my neck, chest, abdomen, and pelvic CT scan. Instead, I was focused on choking down the "mochaccino-flavored" barium, keeping warm in the chilly CT scan room, and convincing the nurse to put the IV into a vein that wasn't hardened from chemo or riddled with scar tissue (an increasingly difficult task after the hundreds of blood draws in the previous two years). With my mission accomplished, I went to work for the rest of the day.

Midafternoon, Dr. Levi called. "Good news is, you still don't have cancer. Bad news is, you have fluid in your pericardial sac. I need you to go to the hospital to be monitored for twenty-four hours. I've already called the ER; they're expecting you. I'm heading out for a long weekend. One of my partners will check in on you tomorrow morning."

Stunned, I took a minute to stare at my beach and my flying girl. Then I shook it off, called Michael, sent a few emails to people who were expecting things from me at work, and hailed a cab.

AT THE ER, Michael and I battled the waves of déjà vu. Here we were, once again, at the ER because I had fluid in my pericardial sac. Here we were, once again, in a private room, dealing with medical students, residents, and attendings. My go-to state in the ER—numbness—was firmly in place. This time, however, it was daylight, so the ER wasn't nearly as entertaining. And this time, I had a long and glorious health history that the doctors could review in order to put me into context. Lydia Slaby: known entity.

In medicine, as in life, people (in this case, doctors) sometimes believe they know what's going on before they actually know what's going on. I walked into the ER on a Friday, two years and two months after my initial cancer diagnosis, as a cancer patient in remission. Therefore, it was very easy for a doctor to look at me and my symptoms and immediately jump to cancer. Because of my sternal wire removal four weeks previously, however, I also walked into the ER that day as a thoracic patient. So, depending on the person (oncologist, cardiologist, thoracic surgeon) and his or her particular focus (cancer, heart disease, virus), my history could paint the present in a seemingly obvious way. This made it very difficult for some doctors to see new symptoms as something other than corroborating an old theory.

The first doctor I saw was the ER attending. She was kind, thoughtful, and no bullshit. After we discussed my history, she looked me straight in the eye and said, "I think it's best for you to know everything that's going on. I don't want you to be unaware of something and then have someone else walk in here assuming you know what they're talking about. Fair?"

Totally. That was a problem when I was first diagnosed in the ER, and it was a horrifying way to learn that I had cancer.

"Your CT scan showed three things," she continued. "One, fluid around your heart, which you already know about. Two, fluid in your lungs. Three, a shadow of unknown density in your anterior mediastinum."

WHAT? My anterior mediastinum was the exact spot where my tumor had lived and died.

Right then and there, my brain stopped being numb and started hyperventilating. My body clenched. I held up my finger to indicate that she needed to stop talking while I closed my eyes and silently took ten long, deep breaths. Mind calmer, body loosened, I opened my eyes and lowered my finger.

The attending didn't miss a beat despite the pause. "The shadow could be fluid or it could be lymph nodes. The radiologist is fairly sure that it's fluid, and Dr. Levi does not seem concerned, but I wanted you to know."

I finally opened my mouth to speak. "How worried should I be about this?"

She nodded her head back and forth, physically equivocating. "I'm not telling you this to make you worried. I'm telling you this to keep you informed. So, only be a little worried."

A little worried. Okay. I can do that. I took another deep breath and settled into "a little worried."

"In the meantime," she went on, "let's talk about the fluid in your pericardial sac and your lungs."

As she kept talking, I kept taking four-count breaths. In-two-three-four . . . out-two-three-four . . . Michael's hand, resting on my ankle, helped soothe me.

My slow counts continued as I got an echocardiogram; as a cardiac fellow explained that there were too many variables to pull the fluid out safely; as I was told by a pair of young thoracic surgeons that there was "no way" the sternal wire removal caused the problem and that I "probably" had cancer again; and as they admitted me back into the cancer wing (because I was a cancer patient in remission) for a twenty-four-hour "wait and see" that made no sense to me.

No decisions were made about what to do with this unwelcome fluid.

Once settled in the cancer wing, I turned toward the evening sun and my husband. We had been working so hard not to have Michael sitting next to me in a hospital bed. To see each other in a new light. To live a new version of our relationship that included passion and laughter and patience and listening. This foray to the hospital was not supposed to be part of that, and my heart clenched. Would we never move past this inexplicable, impossible stage of life?

"Michael, when am I going to be done being a 'cancer patient in remission'?"

He squeezed my foot, face inscrutable. "Hopefully never."

I sighed. "That's not what I mean. This whole thing just seems so unnecessary."

He sat up and kissed my forehead, eyes reflecting my own sadness. "I know."

THE NEXT MORNING, I disconnected my IV and went for a few laps around the floor. The pictures were the same. The rooms where

I had spent so much time two years previously were the same. I hugged a few nurses. And I stood in the sunbeams showering through a large window, floored that this was where I found myself on a beautiful Saturday morning, until I heard Michael's voice floating down the hallway: "She went for a wander. I'm sure she'll be back soon."

I sighed and returned to my room to face whoever wanted me.

It was a double whammy: both the cardiologist from the previous day and one of the members of Dr. Levi's team.

"We figured it would be best to talk to you about this together," one of them said.

"I appreciate the efficiency," I responded. "So, where are we? As of yesterday afternoon you"—nodding to the oncologist—"wanted to remove the fluid and you"—nodding to the cardiologist—"weren't sure it was worth the danger of the procedure. Any updates or conclusions?"

"That just about sums it up," said the other. "We still haven't reached an agreement."

This was the last thing I wanted to be thinking about. The fighter jets from the Chicago Air and Water Show had started thundering over Lake Michigan, distracting me from hospital talk. Feeling like a mediator, I took a deep breath and turned to them. "Give me your arguments and concerns again."

I looked at Michael throughout the conversation, my own internal dialogue shouting through my eyes. *Why the fuck are we the ones who are making this decision? Isn't this their JOB?* Michael, equally flummoxed, held my eyes in understanding.

I could feel—deep-in-my-bones feel, as if someone were

yelling it into my ears—that this whole thing wasn't cancer. I couldn't adequately explain it to Michael, or even to myself, other than saying, "I know I'm not sick again." But I knew it. This knowledge was quiet but visceral. I was still not comfortable with the idea of following my instincts, no matter the volume of their shouting, on medical issues. So this singular voice saying, "I'm fine," was not as powerful as the multiple fear-based voices (mine, Michael's, oncology's) saying, "But maybe not." Living inside that fear, we agreed to remove the fluid early the following week.

We'd gotten used to waiting. Chemo was four months of waiting while the drugs were administered and then waiting to see if they worked. We had waited in waiting rooms, doctor's offices, hospital rooms, pre-op rooms, post-op rooms, infusion suites, at home for phone calls or emails. We had waited just to "give it time." While waiting, we used to have books and phones and computers and tablets and games. But the morning of my fluid-removal procedure, we just had each other. We held hands and told each other stories around what would happen tomorrow—fairy tales around weekend activities . . . horror stories about the latest news of the world . . . love stories about friends and family. The stories that made up our life. Together.

Our storytelling was constantly interrupted by a parade of doctors. First, we met with Dr. Sam, the surgical cardiologist in charge of everything that happened in the cath lab, where cardiologists use robots and tiny tools and screens to do things to your heart. He was about my age, charismatic and considerate. I immediately liked him. A younger resident stood behind him, trailing him quietly like a shadow.

Dr. Sam explained that there was not a tremendous amount

of fluid, and that most of it was behind my heart, making surgery even more complicated. But he remained confident that the procedure could be done safely; otherwise he wouldn't be doing it. Still, there was a chance of possible disaster.

A small part of my mind noticed that he was hedging as much as a lawyer usually does. I wondered what exactly the repercussions of things going sideways looked like. But I was committed to the decision to have the surgery, so I pushed away such thoughts. I had worked hard to get comfortable with whatever might come. He was designated to do the procedure, but in a teaching hospital it is never clear who ends up doing what. Still, I turned to Michael after they left and expressed the hope that Dr. Sam would be the one holding the tools.

Shortly after Dr. Sam left, I met Ted: a short, round nurse wearing one of the warmest smiles I'd ever seen. He wheeled me into the cold cath lab for my procedure, and laid warmed blankets on the metal table before I scooched over from the gurney. Once I was on the table, the well-rehearsed procedures of a surgical suite began. Someone attached my IV to the tubes above my head; someone untied and pulled down my gown while someone else tried to keep me decent with a sterile towel; someone scrubbed my chest with cold Betadine; someone else squirted cold gel under my left breast and shoved the echocardiogram wand into my ribs to display my heart on the monitors surrounding us.

To my relief, Dr. Sam appeared to my right and, showing me the various tools, explained the complicated procedure. He told me they needed me to be in constant communication about feeling anything uncomfortable, so the normal twilight cocktail of painkilling fentanyl and relaxing Versed would not be at full strength. I agreed to these terms, white-knuckling the warm blankets to either side of me.

Then Dr. Sam took a step back, and the younger doctor took the reins.

Someone began pushing the drug combo through my IV, and I started to fade—but as Dr. Sam promised, not enough. I could feel everything. Because of the drugs, it didn't hurt, but my imagination created pain as a companion to what I *could* feel: catheter pushing through skin, then muscle, then whatever else was in my chest cavity, on its way to my heart. I watched the echocardiogram screen as the bright white needle inside my chest slowly approached the blurry, gray, beating shape that was my heart.

The catheter moving through my chest felt like someone was sewing me from the inside out. I could feel tissue separating to make way for it, and I didn't know what level of feeling or pain was a concern, so I just started reporting.

Pressure. "Felt that."

Tear. "Ouch, that actually hurt."

Rubbing. "Feels like sliding."

Poke, poke. "Feels like poking."

Poke, POKE. Tear. "That really feels like poking. Okay, now it's really hurting."

Release. "Okay, that's better."

Dr. Sam paid attention to each of my reports and would correct the other doctor with minute suggestions, their eyes still glued to the screen. Sometimes, Dr. Sam would respond, "More drugs," and I would get a little hazier for a moment.

A couple of times, Ted's face appeared alongside my head, above all of the equipment, as he stroked my forehead, crooning, "Not much longer now, you're doing great."

I tried not to cry. I kept the blankets in a death grip.

Suddenly, there was a flurry of activity on my right. Ted stepped in to clean me up, and a few minutes later I was wheeled back to the recovery room.

Michael jumped up, kissing my forehead and finding my hand. "How you doing?"

I looked up my husband's face, blinking ferociously and hoping he knew what I meant to tell him: how much I loved him for being there, for always being there.

Ted responded for me. "She did great. A little drugged, but that happens. It should clear up in about an hour." He settled me in and left.

I turned my face to Michael, overcome with gratitude for his physical presence, his deep, soothing voice, and his concern. I was having a hard time finding my voice, but I managed to whisper, "I love you. Thank you for being here."

"Of course, Monkey Brain. Nowhere else I'd rather be." He smiled gently.

My mouth twitched up at the corner. I was amused and grateful for his lie.

Not wanting to miss my return from surgery, Michael had waited to take a much-needed bathroom break. As soon as he left, I felt a wave of nausea. I tried to speak, but found no voice. I tried to hit the nurse button, but couldn't raise my arms. I broke out in a cold sweat as my vision narrowed. I was alone. Then I was gone.

WHEN I CAME BACK, the room was crowded with gray and blurry people. Michael was by my left ear, slapping my face gently, calling my name. My fingers and toes tingled lightly. Everyone was staring at the blood pressure monitor behind my head. I had no capacity for emotion, for evaluation. If I had, I would have been petrified.

"What's going on?" I asked in a whisper.

"Your blood pressure crashed," Michael responded from above my head, fingers lingering on my cheek. "It's just come back up to about fifty over thirty, but it was down to forty over twenty a few seconds ago."

People flurried in and out of the room, hooking up new saline bags, pushing new drugs into my IV. Everyone watched the blood pressure monitor. I felt the cuff squeeze my right upper arm. As it released, the entire room took a collective deep breath.

Dr. Sam appeared at my feet. "Well done," he said, patting my foot.

"What's going on?" I asked again. My voice was back and my vision had begun to clear.

"I'm fairly sure that we perforated your heart, and that you're in the process of bleeding out. We're working to get your blood pressure up and steady enough so we can take you back into the cath lab to relieve the pressure on your heart."

Michael was pale, staring at the blood pressure monitor and squeezing my shoulder. I knew he'd heard everything.

Everyone stood in my room for what felt like hours, staring at the blood pressure machine. Once every ten seconds, the cuff would squeeze my right arm and everyone would hold their breath while it released. Someone stayed on my right wrist, tracking my pulse. Someone else sponged my face off. Michael had moved to the foot of the bed and was holding on to my big toe through the blanket. Ted kept coming in and out of the room; he had other patients, but he wouldn't leave me. Dr. Sam was holding my left wrist, alternatively looking at me and the machine.

"Your color is better. How are you feeling?" he asked.

"I'm not sweaty or lightheaded anymore." I picked up my right arm and moved it around, which I thought was success. "I mean, don't ask me to get up and go for a jog, but otherwise I think I'm fine."

"Okay, I think we can do this now."

BACK INTO THE cold room. Three people lifted the sheet and placed me on the metal table. No fancy scooching—not for the girl who was bleeding out. This time, nobody was worried about my decency. Dr. Sam whipped off my gown while someone scrubbed down my chest again. I could see a few medical students gawking through the window from whatever room was on the other side. A much older doctor walked in.

"Where are we?" he asked Dr. Sam. They exchanged medical words.

The older doctor was the epitome of emotionless crisis management. He could have been one of the partners at my law firm. But Dr. Sam was none of that. He was in agony—as his fingers worked a practiced magic with a scalpel and tubing over my right groin, he kept glancing at me, and his eyes couldn't hide his sadness, regret, and determination to fix this disaster.

He finished whatever he had been doing and came up closer to my head. "How you doing?"

I wanted to help him, so I smiled and didn't tell him how frightened I was. "I'm beginning to have trouble taking a deep breath, but I'm assuming you know that."

"Yes, that's to be expected. What we're doing here should help." His fingers were moving somewhere else, checking something, while his eyes stayed on mine.

"What are we doing here?" I was in danger of a full-blown panic attack, but his gaze kept me grounded.

"We're putting in a drain to pull out the blood that is pouring out of your heart."

I didn't know how to respond, so I just looked at him. His look of strain was intense and jarring.

The echocardiogram lady squirted goo on her wand and shoved it back under my left breast and hard against my ribs. *I'm going to have the worst bruise there,* I thought.

"We're going to keep the drugs to a minimum again," Dr. Sam reported.

I took as deep a breath as I could. It wasn't very successful. "Okay." I mentally braced myself for round two.

This time, Dr. Sam stepped forward with the catheter and the older doctor stood behind him. More parting of flesh, more parting of tissue, more unpleasant tearing sensations from inside my chest. This time, I stared at the ceiling and waited for them to be done. My hands, remarkably relaxed, lay across my belly. Someone had put another warm towel across my pelvis, and Ted once again stood by my head. I have no idea how long we all stayed like this.

"Okay," Dr. Sam said, taking a deep breath as he stood back from me.

I looked down and saw a bag of blood lying on my chest. The older doctor clapped Dr. Sam on the back and walked out of the room. He never said a single word to me.

I focused on my body. "Why is there a bag of blood lying on my chest?" I found its warm weight slightly unnerving.

"That's your blood, and it's draining out of your pericardial sac. We're having a hard time keeping the drain from clotting off, but it should do for the next few hours. Please try not to move. How are you doing?" Dr. Sam had moved down a foot and was leaning over my right wrist, where he started doing something else with a scalpel and tubing.

I took as deep a breath as I could (not very) and assessed myself. Then I stopped. Lying to both of us seemed to be the best option. "I'm okay."

He gave me a sad smile.

I closed my eyes and imagined my blood was a hot water bottle, letting the weight of it comfort me. After a while, I relaxed enough to let the cumulative impact of all the drugs and surgeries pull me under.

I FELT MICHAEL'S lips brush against my forehead. "Hey, sweetie," he whispered. "They need to move you."

I opened my eyes and saw a dark room filled with hospital staff. My sheet was lifted and moved onto the new bed, and then the room emptied except for the nurse who circled me, checking all of my tubes (which seemed to be multiplying) and hanging them where they needed hanging.

I learned that I was in the cardiac ICU while the doctors were trying to figure out what to do with me. I could hear voices rumbling in the hallway.

Every now and again, the pressure in my chest would build up and I would tell the nurse that I was having a hard time breathing. She would pop her head into the hallway, and Dr. Sam and Michael would come in. Dr. Sam would lean over my chest, turn a little valve near the bag of my warm blood, and the pressure would release. The third time this happened, the pressure didn't fade.

Dr. Sam looked at the bag. "It's clotted off. We're not going to be able to get any more blood out of your chest this way. How bad is your breathing?"

"Um, I can still breathe, if that's what you mean. It's just"—I searched for the right word, communing with my lungs—"tight."

"Okay. Tight is okay."

He walked back out of the room to join the mumbling voices in the hallway. I nodded at his retreating back, too miserable and confused and drugged to say anything in response. Michael took my hand, kissed it, and waited with me.

A new doctor walked in, and I immediately identified him as a surgeon. There's something in the way that surgeons hold themselves—inconceivably confident but also not quite able to meet your eyes. And when he introduced himself as a cardiac surgeon, I erupted into pure, unfiltered anger. I was completely prone on the bed, only able to move my head, my left arm, and my left leg, but that didn't matter. "Get out," I ordered him.

"I'm sorry?"

"If you are here to tell me that you have to cut me open again to solve this disaster, I will end you." My rage tinted him red and gave him little devil horns.

My left hand was still lying across my belly holding Michael's. His fingers moved inside it, trying to get some breathing room. I loosened my grip a bit and took a tight breath, trying not to burst into tears.

The surgeon made a valiant attempt to look me in the eyes. He plowed through my glare with lots of words. "Let's start over, shall we? My name is Tripp Shuman, and I'm sorry that we're meeting under these conditions. For the past few hours, about a dozen of us in the hallway have been trying to figure out how to solve your problem. The last thing any of us want to do is cut you open again. I know you've already had a sternotomy and a thymectomy, and I know you just had the wires removed and the scar revised. But here's the situation."

Dr. Shuman held up his left hand in a fist and covered it with his right hand.

"Your heart"—he waved his left fist—"is completely surrounded by a blood clot that is about two centimeters thick." Then he waved his right hand. "The pericardial sac kept the blood that came out of the hole in your right ventricle in the immediate vicinity of your heart, which is great news for the rest of your chest but really bad news for your heart. It's this pressure from the blood clot that is causing your shortness of breath, in the same way that you had the shortness of breath from the excess fluid."

He stopped talking, giving me a moment to say something. I nodded for him to go on, so furious that I had no words.

"We're pretty sure that the actual hole, which is about half the diameter of a pencil, has clotted off at this point and is probably healing as we speak. Heart muscle heals incredibly fast because it's bathed in blood. So that's the good news. The bad news is, the blood surrounding your heart is mostly clotted as well, which is why we can't pull it out and into this bag anymore."

He pointed to the warm bag of blood still lying on my chest. Then he explained my two options: One, they could go back into my chest, using scopes and cameras to see what they were doing, and pull out as much of the clot as possible. Two, they could open me up and get a full view of what was happening in my chest, including that dark shadow from the CT scan, and then clean up my heart with no danger of perforating it again.

"But we can't, in good conscience, let you leave the hospital until I remove that clot," he finished.

My anger, so quick to flare, was already burning out, stunned at the barrage of information and giving way to resignation. He knew everything and had already preemptively answered all of my questions. With the impossible knowledge that I would soon be back on the surgical table, my anger dissipated and I simply broke. I started crying—snot, tears, the whole thing.

Dr. Shuman said some words to Michael and backed out of the room.

"I don't want to do this again," I choked out. "Please don't make me do this again."

Michael was quiet.

My mind spun in agony for a few moments until I heard Dr. Sam's discreet footsteps. His appearance brought my focus back to the present situation in one beat of my abused heart.

"I know. I know. I don't have a fucking choice. Let's crack open my chest and solve this goddamn problem." My voice was even and defeated.

Dr. Sam quietly turned and left.

"Do you want to call your parents?" asked Michael.

I actually laughed, one small breathy *ha*. "Not even a little bit. I'll call Corinna. Isn't it her job as older sister to run interference?"

Corinna answered, and I caught her up on everything that had happened since the CT scan, including the fact that I was now lying in the ICU with a hole in my heart. Dr. Sam reentered the room in the middle of my explanation.

"Are you joking?" she asked, almost laughing. "Is this a true story?"

"Cross my heart."

"Very funny. So, now what?"

I caught her up on the plan for the evening's procedure, imagining Dr. Shuman using a tiny, red shop vacuum to suck up all the blood. This image somehow kept my panic at bay.

"Do me a favor." Corinna's voice came through clearly on the speakerphone. "Don't die tonight."

Dr. Sam's head dropped as if he'd been punched in the stomach. He turned and walked back out of the room.

"Corinna, you just made my doctor cry."

"Good."

I remembered Dr. Sam's kind, reassuring gaze during the second procedure and immediately rose to his defense. "No, he's a nice guy. Nobody meant to poke a hole in my heart. Besides, I'm pretty sure a resident poked a hole in my heart, and he's taking the blame for it."

Her response was visceral and colorful and filled with righteous anger and love, and it did far more to comfort me than my hot water bottle of blood. We kept up our words of comfort for each other until Dr. Shuman walked back into my room with Michael behind him.

"I have to go," I told my sister. "I'm assuming the surgeon who just walked into my room wants to tell me more horrible details that I don't want to know about how they have to crack open my chest again."

"Have fun with that. Good luck. And I love you." Her voice echoed as Michael reached over my shoulder and ended the call.

I leaned into the love in her voice, using it to give me the strength to turn back to Dr. Shuman. "I love you too," I whispered to the room.

DISMEMBERMENT

EXTRAORDINARY CHANGE—physical, mental, emotional, spiritual—can happen in moments of extreme trauma. The shamanic world describes it as *dismemberment*—the "coming apart" of trauma that then allows for reformation, or *re-memberment*. In indigenous traditions, the process of dismemberment and re-memberment cleans up current- or past-life karma and discards anything that is not helpful for the present or the future: emotions, emotional memories, muscle memory, energetic residue, scars. Traditionally, priests, shamans, medicine men, or indigenous healers help a person through the dismembering process, because otherwise one is left adrift. As I felt after chemo. As I felt after my thymus surgery. And as I felt most powerfully after my heart surgery.

When I woke up again in a darkened room, my eyes refused to open. I couldn't breathe. Air was pumping in and out of my lungs, but I had no control over it. In response, I tried breathing through my nose and immediately gagged. Something was in my mouth. My arms jerked up reflexively to try and pull out whatever it was, but something soft bound my wrists to my sides. Adrenaline flooded my body, and I tried to fight my way out of the restraints, but the rest of my body was weighed down by something. I couldn't shake my head.

I felt two hands come down on my shoulders, and heard Michael's voice making soothing noises from my right. "Sweetie, calm down. You're in recovery. You still have a breathing tube in."

Enough of the surgical anesthetic was out of my system to let me believe I could breathe on my own, but I wasn't awake enough for anything else. I could only comprehend two things: being trapped in some kind of physical hell and Michael's hand rubbing mine.

The hell stayed with me as I learned about this toothbrush-like thing stuck in my mouth. If I breathed through my nose, I choked and my body would seize in reaction. I could breathe through my mouth, but it wasn't entirely under my own control—which was a different kind of hell, though at least it kept me breathing. I started taking deep breaths through my mouth, working with whatever was controlling part of my breathing. I was so tired and drugged, though, that every few breaths I would forget what I was doing and try to breathe through my nose. Then the whole thing would fall apart. Tears made trails down the side of my face and started to pool in my ears.

"Lydia," said a new voice, "You can do it. Just focus on breathing through your mouth. In . . . out . . . in . . . out . . ."

My breathing slowed.

"There you go. Well done. Now, I need to test how strong your lungs are. When I stop the machine that's helping you breathe, you need to breathe in as hard as you can so I can measure your lung strength. It will be really uncomfortable, but I can't remove the breathing tube until I know you have enough power to breathe on your own."

My body found my eyelids at last, and I opened them to see Michael, smiling. "Hi," he whispered softly. He looked like I felt: exhausted, dazed, and about a hundred years old.

I squeezed his hand.

The new voice belonged to a man in his twenties or thirties, leaning over me from my left. "I'm Sean, your ICU nurse. Can you move your head?"

It took a few minutes, but at last I gave Sean a small nod. Exhausted from the effort, my eyes drifted closed, and I dozed off.

When I woke up again, a few minutes or a few hours later, I had forgotten my hard-earned knowledge about breathing through my mouth, so I flailed against my manacles and torturous toothbrush until Sean's voice cut through my panic again. "In . . . out . . . in . . . out . . ."

Michael squeezed my right hand, and the adrenaline dissipated.

"Welcome back."

I pointed my chin in Sean's direction to let him know that I'd heard him.

"Let's start the process of testing your lung power, okay? I'll count to three, and on three I'll turn off the machine, and you have to breathe in through your mouth as hard as you can, okay?"

I nodded.

"One . . ."

Breathe in.

"Two . . ."

Breathe out.

"Three."

I made the movement to breathe in but couldn't. The sensation was familiar, like when my sister used to put her hand over the top of my snorkel tube. I was sucking, but nothing was coming in.

"You're doing a great job," Sean cheered. "Just breathe harder. You can do it!"

I tried harder, but my lungs were burning. To compensate, my body switched to my nose without asking my brain first if it was a good idea, and I started choking again.

Sean turned the machine back on while I was jerking at my wrist manacles.

The tears started again. *Why are they making me do this? I can* BREATHE, *which is why I keep choking. So why the hell are they torturing me with a test?* My continuous choking and failed coughing had irritated my throat, and it was beginning to feel like someone had rubbed sandpaper down my trachea.

Michael's thumb made fast circles on my right palm. "Are you okay, sweetie?"

I shook my head no, snot running out of my nose. I tried to sniff it back in and started choking again.

Sean wiped my nose with something soft and put his hand on my left shoulder. "I can't take the tube out until you hit thirty on this machine. That last time you made it to 25, which is great. So next time you just need to try a little bit harder. Do you want a break?"

I shook my head no. I needed to get this shit over and done as fast as possible. All thoughts were scattered. The pain and constant focus on breathing were the only things I could think about, and I needed them, a visceral, painful need, to be over.

"Okay. One . . ." *In.*

"Two . . ." *Out.*

"Three."

I tried again, but my lungs started burning even faster this time. I kept sucking and sucking and clamping Michael's hand even harder in response to encouragement from both men, and then I gave up.

The air came back on, and I dozed off.

It felt like I tried a half dozen more times, dozing off between attempts, for what seemed to be three or four hours. Every now and then, I would start choking or coughing, which would invoke a full body spasm.

Finally, Michael had enough. I don't remember what he said to Sean, but in response, Sean told me to take a deep breath in and, as I breathed out for a count of five, pulled out the toothbrush tube.

I mouthed the words *thank you* to my torturer and immediately fell back asleep as he freed my wrists from their fabric handcuffs.

I thought cancer was the most horrible, life-changing diagnosis possible. Right up until I had entirely unnecessary emergency heart surgery.

WHEN I WOKE up again, I had the energy to open my eyes. Michael was asleep to my right, draped over the bed railing, his hand still holding mine. Sean was on my left, squeezing some kind of sponge over a small bowl. He ran it down my left arm, scrubbing various bits and pieces. This must have been what awakened me.

We had a quiet exchange while I used the sponge bath to inventory my body. A huge bandage covered my entire groin area. I had some kind of line coming out of my right forearm. A tube coming out of the right side of my neck. An enormous bandage between my breasts, from my throat down to my diaphragm, covering the surgical site and the entrance wounds to four drains, which exited my body between my lowest ribs. Various heart monitor sticky pads were strategically placed around the bandage.

Michael had woken up while Sean was cleaning my right leg and was watching the process.

"What time is it?" I whispered hoarsely, my throat chafed from the breathing tube.

"Around four thirty. You got out of surgery around midnight and woke up about an hour ago."

"An *hour* ago?" I would have bet everything I owned and then some that I had been dozing on and off for at least five to six hours. The breathing tube fiasco, which I had been so convinced took longer than the entire *Lord of the Rings* movie trilogy, happened over only about forty-five minutes.

I looked at my shattered husband. "Please go back to sleep," I begged him.

Michael didn't need asking twice. He curled up in the chair next to my bed and fell asleep again in seconds.

I raised the head of the bed about a foot so I could see around me a little more successfully, verified with Sean that he was done with me for the moment, and went back to sleep myself.

When I woke again, soft morning light was filtering through the shaded window. Michael was gently kissing my forehead, explaining that he was heading home for a nap. Elizabeth, recruited to stay with me, was standing behind him. As her voice pattered along, telling me stories of her new beau, calmly pulling me out of my reality, I did a mental inventory of my torn-apart body. I could open my eyes, but it was exhausting, so I didn't. My body felt weighted down and swollen. I twitched my leg muscles to see if they worked, and a lightning bolt of fire shot down my right leg in response.

The day passed in a haze of removing tubes: central line, blood pressure monitor, catheter, two of four drains. Elizabeth was a quiet, steady presence. Doctors came and went.

First was Dr. Shuman. "You're up! Well done."

"Fuck you," I grumbled with my eyes closed. My rage had dissipated, but I was still firmly aware that I had just had unnecessary open-heart surgery.

He started poking at bandages and listening to my lungs and heart while I asked questions. I was swollen, and he told me this was causing the fire in my right leg. "It's because we put you on bypass last night."

"You did what now?"

Apparently after the first chest-opening surgery, one of my major veins fused to the inside of my sternum. Dr. Shuman knew this because when he opened me up again, the vein tore apart. They had put me on bypass for twenty to thirty minutes while he repaired the damage to the vein.

I breathed quietly during his description of this latest near-death experience, my hundredth or so of the past twenty-four hours, deciding that nothing else could surprise me that day. Then he gave me a pat on the head and walked out of the recovery room.

Elizabeth chuckled. "Did he just pat you on the head?"

"Well, I did threaten to end him yesterday," I confessed, "so I feel like our relationship has progressed."

Michael later told me that when Dr. Shuman had completed the surgery around midnight, he came out of the surgical suite and his face had gotten a little soft. "You know," he had revealed, "your wife has the most beautiful heart I've ever held." Michael, stretched to the brink, was reduced to tears on his waiting room chair.

"Dr. Shuman is the one who fixed the problem," Elizabeth responded to me now. "Why didn't you threaten to end the one who created it instead?"

"Because Dr. Sam was so nice. And besides, he didn't do it. A goddamn resident did." *Fucking students.*

As if on cue, Dr. Sam walked in. "How are you doing?" he asked.

I gave a small shrug, delighted to discover that at least this one movement didn't hurt. "I just had heart surgery, so that's how I'm doing. But that shrug didn't hurt, so . . . progress! How are you?"

He shook his head sadly. "I can't believe you're asking me that question in light of everything that's happened in the last day."

I took a breath, picking my next words carefully, letting compassion drive the choice. "Mistakes happen. I get it. Please don't let this weigh on you."

He stared at me, gaping. "I don't know how to respond to that."

I smiled. "You can respond by not letting it happen to anyone else, okay?"

He continued to stare at me, tears glistening in his eyes. A moment later, he shook himself out of wherever his brain had taken him and asked me to lean forward so he could listen to my heart and lungs.

Later, Michael told me that while I was in the ICU, as the various surgeons and doctors discussed my bleeding heart, Dr. Sam refused to leave my side. His job was over, but he wouldn't leave. His dedication and compassion—let alone my own need to move forward—deserved my forgiveness.

"HEY THERE, Sweetbreads."

At this greeting, I practically burst into tears on the spot. It was Dr. McLean, his face so friendly and kind and suffused with worry.

Dr. McLean had starting calling me this shortly after removing my own "sweetbreads"—I think he meant to say the all-purpose "sweetheart" instead. I found it hilarious and endearing, as did he, but he begged me not to tell the hospital administrators. It wasn't exactly professional.

"Hi," I responded.

He sat cautiously at the foot of my bed. "I heard you had a rough night."

"That's an understatement." I picked up both arms as if I were Exhibit A. "How do I get square with this?" I explained that I didn't want to blame anyone for the unnecessary heart surgery—and that at the same time, I kind of wanted to blame someone. Dr. Sam, for letting the resident screw up the initial procedure. The resident, for screwing up. Dr. Shuman, for failing to meet my eyes when he had to come in and clean up the mess. Dr. Levi, for being the all-knowing wizard behind the curtain, pushing the surgery because of what she saw in my scan. The whole thing really sucked.

Dr. McLean took a deep breath and sat down near my feet on the bed. "You might as well blame me. I'm the one who gave you an unnecessary thymectomy last year."

I had a running shit list, but hadn't considered adding him to it. My left eyebrow twitched in response.

"Well, it turns out your tumor was completely dead, so the thymectomy was unnecessary," Dr. McLean continued. "As a result, you had unnecessary sternal wires, which you then wanted removed because they were uncomfortable, which then led to the current situation." He spread his hands to indicate where we were and all that had happened.

My brain clicked on, vindication coursing through my chest. "Ah. So you've decided that removing the sternal wires caused all of this?"

"We can't think of any other reason. Dr. Shuman didn't see anything in your chest cavity where the CT scan showed a shadow, so it was probably just fluid that ran out the minute he opened you up."

For a moment, I chewed on everything he'd said. "If I start thinking all this was unnecessary, I'm going to jump out a window."

"Which is why your instincts are telling you to just take it all in stride. You, more than anyone else on this floor right now, know how much of medicine is art, not science. I've been doing this for too long and have seen too much to claim that doctors are infallible. We're human." He shrugged. "We do the best we can, but none of us are God." He paused and chuckled. "Despite what some of the younger surgeons believe."

I looked at him and took a deep, shuddering breath. "Okay."

He smiled. "Make sure you breathe like that as much as possible. You don't want your lungs getting crunchy. How are you doing on tube removal?"

"I think I'm mostly done, but I still have all four drains in."

He stood up. "Okay, you work on getting those down to two, and I'll go throw some patients out of recovery so you can get up there this afternoon. Deal?"

"Deal." I smiled and blinked back tears as Dr. McLean patted my leg and moved off.

THE REST OF the day passed in a haze. Rust-colored liquid slowly dripped into my four drains, and in due course, the nurse removed the two that filled the slowest. Michael returned with pillows and slippers. Eighteen hours after I had open-heart surgery, they sent me up to recovery.

As the hours and days ticked by, my friends showed up with forced smiles and tried not to harbor too much wrath for the hospital, Dr. Levi, or Dr. Sam. I kept giving my same practiced speech: "Doctors can't apologize for messing up, because of malpractice suits. I refuse to contribute my own condemnation to a system that prevents the humans who work inside it from making amends. Besides, what are they going to do, reverse time? This is not a problem that money can solve, and I will not ruin Dr. Sam's life."

Dr. Sam kept checking on me, looking like Eeyore. We kept feeling each other out with the tentative *How are you?* And I kept reminding him that mistakes happen and he needed to forgive himself for it. I tried to make sure he understood that I knew his continued presence was the only apology I would get from him, and that I forgave him. All of this is hard to do when you can't legally say the words.

Not for the first time, I cursed the insanity created by my chosen profession.

Ted the cardiac nurse showed up once and gave me a hug. We chatted for a while about nothing much while he snuck subtle peeks at my bandages. Then he left, wiping his eyes when he thought I could no longer see him.

I WAS DISCHARGED from the hospital on Sunday, four and a half days after heart surgery. That Monday morning, I received a text message from Dr. Levi: THE BIOPSY OF THE FLUID REMOVED FROM YOUR PERICARDIAL SAC SHOWED NO SIGN OF CANCER!

I stared at this statement, slowly reminding myself of the reason why all this had happened—and feeling that her exclamation point was a bit much. I typed out my response: THIS IS THE MOST ANTICLIMACTIC TEXT MESSAGE I'VE EVER RECEIVED. BUT THANKS. SEE YOU NEXT WEEK. Then I threw my phone across the room.

Luckily for my phone, it landed just a few feet away on the foot of the bed. My arms still weren't working quite right.

EXACTLY TWO WEEKS after the day of the heart debacle, I had follow-up X-rays and appointments with all of my doctors. Spreading my arms wide for the X-ray hurt like a bitch, but I was trying to get off of opiates, so I gritted my teeth and took a steadying breath. Dr. Shuman's nurse made me cough while pushing against my sternum and examined the eight healing incisions scattered across my torso, created by her boss. My GP took one look at me and suggested I stay out of the hospital for a little bit. I chuckled weakly.

The hardest conversation was with Dr. Levi. I had not seen her at all since my open-heart surgery, because she'd been out of town during the whole fiasco. She crept into the exam room, hiding behind my chart, and sat heavily down on the chair with a rueful grin.

I didn't smile back. My love for this woman and everything she had done for me was enduring, but that day it was taking a bit of a break.

I spoke first. "Well, now that we've actually looked inside my chest and we know for a fact that the shadow on the CT scan was not cancer, I think I'm done with my semi-annual CT scans." My voice was level, a fact I noted with no small amount of pride. But my patience was running out as quickly as the Tylenol I'd taken four hours previously.

Dr. Levi kept a safe distance from where I sat. "I'm so sorry you went through this."

Still quietly angry, but composed, I responded with practicality. "Well, I did, and it's done. So let's talk about what we're going to do moving forward."

To her credit, she stayed calm and offered her regrets again. Then my blood work appeared on the screen, showing severely low red blood counts and depleted white blood counts.

My equilibrium fell to the wayside. Before this gigantic mess happened, my counts had been rebounding. "Are you fucking kidding me?" I exclaimed.

Dr. Levi suggested that I have a blood transfusion and start pounding iron supplements.

"Sure. And *no more scans*. I'm *not going through this again*." My voice was forceful but controlled, yet she twitched as if I had yelled.

As I gathered myself up to leave her office, heading for the blood clinic, she suggested that we see each other again in three months, and we could talk about it then. I told her what she could do with that idea.

DISMEMBERMENT. Despite their kindness and concern, none of my doctors could help put Humpty Dumpty completely back together again. In modern medicine, we have forgotten about *re-memberment*, about the need to heal the body on multiple levels once it is damaged. Doctors have replaced priests in many respects—we turn to them for the miracle of saving our lives. But they haven't been trained in spiritual healing, so problems arise when the doctor saves the physical body and ignores its connection to the mind, emotions, spirit, and energy.

The most obvious example of this is the danger that stress presents in our body. Heart disease arises from a combination of poor diet choices and stress, a mental affliction. Given that it is caused by more than pure physiology, we need to recover from it in more than just physical terms—through a multipronged approach. Mental health, spiritual calm, and emotional stability are just as important as whatever diet is suggested and any pills that are prescribed.

When one accepts this idea of marrying the physical with the spirit, mind, emotions, and energy, the concept of surgery appears both simpler and more complicated. A surgeon cuts; a body is damaged and then stitched back together. But if indeed we are a pulsing energetic field in addition to skin and muscle and bone, the scalpel has cut more than the body. It has eviscerated the energetic field in which the body resides. Some theories, primarily in Eastern medicine—like acupuncture—hold that damage to this energetic field causes damage to the body. Body woes can be solved only if the energy is healed.

So how can the body ever truly come back together if the energetic field has been ignored? Why must the power of our mind and our energy be sidelined in favor of the physical miracle of our body? Where are the stitches to help reintegrate energy and flesh? When is the surgeon trained to recognize the importance of healing both? This is where we need to introduce re-memberment in the modern surgical suite.

If surgeons were trained to understand that every cut they make is also gutting the body energetically and spiritually, both the patient and her body would be in much better condition. And let's not forget the surgeon. What untold damage befalls the surgeon, as an agent of dismemberment without the training and wisdom to fully understand the repercussions? Dr. Shuman's inability to meet my eye. Dr. Sam's pain. In this respect, the modern decoupling of medicine from faith has done both giver and taker a tremendous disservice. This cataclysmic crack in one's psyche is akin to torture—a fragmenting mind-body experience I had dreamed about countless times.

One way a human reacts to physical torture is to experience a loss of time, a phenomenon so well documented that it has its own word: *duration*, as in "the experience went on for a duration." In moments during my time of so-called healing, I was living entirely in the present, to the point of losing any concept of past or future. My brain couldn't help me escape this scenario because my mind, like everyone's, lives in the past or the future. My mind couldn't pull me out of a "now" that was so immediate and eviscerating.

My present was created by the trauma of dismemberment—by pharmaceuticals (the day of my bony pain during chemo), by surgical error (the failure to stabilize my heart as blood poured out of a hole in my right ventricle), and by procedure (the breathing tube disaster). At what point did I really consent to all this? At what point did I agree that the ends justified the means? At what point did my doctors consent to address only one part of their patients? At what point did I become so disconnected from my own body that this dismembering process became okay?

In an ideal universe, as these traumatic moments occurred, someone trained in holistic healing would sweep in to help clean up the mess—for both patient and doctor. Dr. Sam, as far as I could tell, needed help as much as I did.

I wasn't living in an ideal universe. I knew from the moment I saw Dr. Levi and realized that I loathed this woman who I also loved so deeply and permanently, that for both our sakes, I had to rethink how to approach my own health.

I was sick to death of almost being killed to save my life. I was frustrated and infuriated and disgusted that no road map existed for my recovery. My dreams and my instincts were telling me at last that I needed something more than to *go back*. I needed to begin the process of re-membering.

DEATH

WHEN I WAS DIAGNOSED with my version of non-Hodgkin's lymphoma, the conversation moved so quickly from *You have cancer* to *We know how to deal with this particular version of it* that I never truly thought about whether I was going to die. One doctor even went so far as to tell me that he'd rather have my cancer than diabetes. "Sure, it's an annoying six months," he quipped, "but then you're done."

My parents, however, couldn't help but worry about my impending demise. Neither could my sister. Or all of my friends. Or Michael. The possibility was always there, lurking in the background.

Cancer, in our society, equals death. This is what we all understand, whether from our grandparents who died from some form or another of this virulent disease, or from the bald, emaciated actor reaching out from the bed toward a loved one before gasping her last breath as the family collapses around her in dramatized agony. Susan Sontag noticed this phenomenon with frustration forty years ago, when she wrote *Illness as Metaphor*. Got cancer? Nice knowing you.

Otherwise, we don't really talk about it. If you have cancer and you aren't on the brink of death, your experience is largely invisible. This is how I found myself in an unfriendly land with no maps.

Throughout the entire experience, chemo sat squarely in the middle of my consciousness. Death, meanwhile, was never on my mind. Not until I was a week out of chemo and in the process of deciding how much energy I had to spend on recovering from it. That's when Michael and I heard the news that his stepbrother had collapsed in his kitchen while making breakfast for his two sons. It was a heart attack. He never recovered.

Michael has three parents: his dad, his mom, and his stepmom, who has been in his life since he was nine. She is such a vital part of his life that I tend to think that I have two mothers-in-law. With his father's second marriage, Michael acquired his only siblings. And it was his older brother, Zach, whose heart felled him at the age of forty-four.

My blood counts had rebounded just in time, and we made the trip to a lovely, remote part of Northern California for a funeral that should have taken place at least forty years later. There, we celebrated Zach's life and did what we could to support those who were most affected by his death: Zach's wife, two sons, sister, and mother.

Absent any useful directive that might guide my way, I had compartmentalized my sister's cancer in two pieces: the part I thought about (helping her through chemo and recovery and all attendant challenges) and the part I refused to think about (the possibility of her death). But neither my experience nor my imagination did anything to prepare me for the day of this funeral for a man whom I had never even met in person.

The burial took place on a clear, crisp, autumn afternoon, in the shadow of undulating brown hills. We stood quietly as the pastor spoke the final official words to send Zach off to his next spot, wherever that might be. As the pastor's voice faded, the contained grief of the family was finally expressed, and the fifty-odd people in attendance witnessed a wife's loss. Her keening sobs cut straight through me, and I began to cry.

Michael wrapped his arms around me and pressed his face against my cheek, and both of us held each other with quiet desperation. I was not quite aware that what I was feeling—the reaction to another person's sorrow—was a reflection of my husband's agony during my treatment. This was a partner's pain. This was Michael's pain. And for as long as the widow wept, not a soul moved. All of our hearts melted and screamed along with her.

When at last she quieted, the crowd shook itself and began the slow walk back to the cars.

But Michael didn't move. I stood with him, wondering. After a long while, I turned into his hug and held him, feeling his hot tears land on my bald head, realizing that some of those tears were for me.

UNTIL I WAS diagnosed with cancer, death and I were rare dance partners.

My mother's father died when I was in second grade. I didn't like him. He gave slobbery kisses and creeped me out. So his being gone was actually a bit of a relief. I felt sad for my mother, who was clearly upset by the whole thing, but I didn't feel sad for myself, and I certainly didn't miss him.

When I was in fourth grade, a friend was killed in a car accident. He was sweet and funny and cute, and I don't think any of us really understood what happened. But after a few weeks, I began to miss him. That's when I realized that I would never see him again. I didn't have any way to process the emotions that come with this dreadful, sudden awareness. That was the worst part; and because it happened long after his death, I felt alone in my sorrow. I was grieving "late" and grieving "wrong."

As I got older and lost my other three grandparents, I began to understand that this emotional lag time is typical for me, and I stopped judging myself for it.

About ten months after my heart surgery—almost three years after the cancer diagnosis—my friend Dan was killed on his third trip to Mount Everest. It was his second attempt at trying to summit the beast; his trip the year before had been cut short when an avalanche killed sixteen and the Sherpas went on strike. This year, a huge earthquake somewhere near Kathmandu had shaken the snow loose on Everest, sending everyone at base camp scrambling for their lives. Dan had suffered a fatal head wound. He was thirty-three, and one of the most alive people I'd ever had the delight in knowing.

As with Zach, the news of Dan's death remained unreal until his memorial service. This time, however, something new happened to me during those few weeks between the news and the ceremony. As expected, I reacted to death with delayed sadness. What I absolutely did not expect to feel was joy.

Michael was predictably stunned by Dan's accident, so I didn't say anything at all about this new emotion peeking up through the haze of mourning. But it was there: a deep, resounding joy. I was happy for Dan. As I watched myself fill with joy, I tried simultaneously to avoid judging myself for it and to understand it. I tried to see where this joy had come from and where it was going. It felt too traitorous to actually indulge myself in the joy, so I stepped back from it and observed it. And I discovered a few things.

Dan had loved life. He had lived it so completely that he often didn't sleep for days. While holding a full-time job, he'd traveled to forty countries in three years, often choosing to interact with the local population at a depth not usually experienced by tourists. He loved adventures and frequently found himself in ridiculous or dangerous or ridiculously dangerous situations—sometimes of his own creation. He was determined to explore his spiritual side. Many of the conversations we'd had focused on our own paths and how they were unfolding. Summiting Everest had been one of his dreams for as long as I'd known him. And he'd died there, doing what he loved in a culture that would help guide his energetic spirit and curious soul along its path. He died brushing the heavens.

I sat with this weird joy for days until I met with Ruth and told her about it, more than a little embarrassed to be happy for my dead friend.

"Am I a terrible person?" I asked her, not for the first time. "Is my psyche broken?"

She laughed. "You're not broken at all. I promise."

After chatting with her and spending some time with both

the emotion and our conversation, I realized that my normal human fear of death had shifted. I had faced death so many times in the previous few years that I no longer feared my inevitable departure. I only feared that it might happen on a hospital bed.

I was happy for Dan, because if that was his moment to go, he died while doing exactly what he loved doing. If we could all be so lucky.

I took these two things along with me—my epiphany in one hand and my joy in the other—to Dan's memorial service. About 150 people met in a vineyard in Napa Valley under the crystal-clear sky of an eight-year drought. There, we ate, drank, laughed, cried, and performed our own private ceremonies of grief and letting go. People had shown up in costume: dinosaurs were preferred, second only to Burning Man outfits. I sat quietly in black and sunglasses. The stories were incredible. The laughter was cathartic.

At the end of the afternoon, a Nepalese monk led the entire group through a traditional Himalayan ceremony intended to pray for safety on Sagarmatha (Everest)—or perhaps it was for safe passage after a trek up the mountain doesn't go as planned. It didn't really matter. His chanting quieted the group and gave me a chance to sit quietly on the ground and connect with Mother Nature and the spirits all around us. Sitting there with my joy in my lap and the chanting and birdsong in my ears, I finally found the space for images to float through my head—some of Dan, some of my own history—and I began to grasp what it means to have a changed relationship with death.

I began to weep. I wept for Dan's life being cut short when Sagarmatha claimed her vibrant sacrifice. I wept for my own body, completely abused and dismembered and changed over the previous three years. I wept for Michael's and my newlywed phase, cut short by anger, frustration, and disease. I wept for Dan's girlfriend, who had lost her person and would never know what the future could have been like with him by her side.

And then I prayed. One of the spiritual traditions in Nepal holds that the most dangerous time for a soul is the forty-nine days after its separation from the body. During that time, the soul says its good-byes and starts searching out its next path. If it is held too tightly by the living, it will stay in order to try and make them feel better, sacrificing its own need to move on to the next plane or reincarnate. So I prayed for Dan to find his next path. I prayed for those still holding on to him to let him go. And I bowed my head in gratitude for my healthy body and for my marriage: both scarred but whole, both seeking vibrancy.

The chanting carried my prayers into the wind, and from my shoulders lifted a weight I hadn't realized I'd been carrying.

AS I LAY in bed for two weeks after my unexpected heart surgery, I contemplated my most recent dismemberment . . . the harrowing months that led up to my cancer diagnosis . . . the disease that effectively stopped my marriage's downward spiral . . . all the bumps and twists and turns that had brought me to the hospital again and again. I reflected on my mind-set, my knowledge, my behavior. In short, I performed a complete inventory of the previous four years.

According to some theories, cancer is a physical manifestation of our shadow-side. If our human body is a miracle of light and energy, rapidly dividing, rapacious cancer cells are the bogeymen who live in the dark. Our body is a balance of healthy and unhealthy, yin and yang, feminine and masculine, light and dark, energy and shadow. Can we survive without abnormal cells? Absolutely. Is it possible for our physical miracles of light and evolution to exist without creating abnormal cells? Probably not. Not if we evolve from ape to human. Not if we grow from maiden to crone. Not if we change over either millennia or the course of a lifetime. Our bodies are constantly producing tiny mistakes alongside millions of pieces of perfection. So why does cancer—these tiny mistakes, these shadows—blossom?

Yes, there are known triggers for the disease: toxins, genetics, general inflammation, stress. But it doesn't strike with any logical pattern. It picks and chooses. Western medicine would say it picks those whose immune systems are weakest or whose time has come—a remarkably metaphysical comment that I've heard from the mouth of more than one doctor. With my data set of precisely two people (me and my sister) plus some smokers I've known, I'm not sure that's true.

Cancer becomes a problem when the cells in our own body reproduce at a rate faster than our immune system can kill them off. It's not an "other" in the way that I tend to classify disease. It's not a bacteria or a virus or a small parasite of a different ilk. It is us. It is me. There is no entity outside of my own physiology to blame. Of everyone my age with my diet and exercise regime and ten years without a cigarette, *I* was the one who got cancer.

Why? I thought as I lay in bed watching Ellie crouch and stalk and wiggle her butt in advance of pouncing on Jake.

Cancer first appears in medical literature around 400 BC

when the physician Hippocrates described it as *karkinos*, from the Greek word for "crab," because that's how a tumor physically appeared to him. He was also the first to describe the human body in terms of the delicate balance of the four cardinal fluids called *humors*: blood, black bile, yellow bile, and phlegm. In a healthy body, these humors are held in perfect balance. Excess of one or more fluids would upset this balance and cause illness.

Claudius Galen, a surgeon and philosopher born in 130 AD, took Hippocrates' humoral theory of the body and set about assigning each illness to a humor. Inflammation went with red blood. Pustules and lymph, notable for their white coloring, went with phlegm. Jaundice coupled with yellow bile. Galen reserved the malevolent, oily, viscous black bile for only two ailments: the disease of cancer and the dis-ease of depression. He proposed that black bile trapped in a specific place in the body became cancer. As bile was systematic, so was the cancer that would result from this dark clot.

History progressed. After the humoral theories were disproved, the fight against cancer became a fight against a single, solid tumor that could be caught or controlled by increasingly horrific, radical surgeries. It wasn't until the 1940s that Sidney Farber, the father of modern chemotherapy, floated the idea that a systemic chemical attack could kill cancer. This idea wasn't widely accepted until the late 1960s. In so many ways, our modern theory—that cancer is a systemic disease that requires systemic treatment—is still very young.

This is true, but incomplete. Our modern approach of systemic chemotherapy only addresses the physical side. Cancer is so much more than that.

If we humans are light and energy and hope and vibrancy, doesn't our shadow-side deserve more than simple chemical warfare? What if the response to cancer requires not only physical intervention, but also a complete process of stripping back how the shadow became so powerful? What if treatment and recovery require deep emotional and spiritual and mental evaluation, support, and healing? What if the process requires us to get truly naked, not just with our cells but with everything that makes us who we are?

Which brings us back 1,900 years, to Galen and his black bile. Without electron microscopes or gene sequencing or any of the other fancy equipment and processes that litter modern research institutions, Galen understood something fundamental: that cancer, although it sometimes only manifests as a single, potentially operable tumor, is at its heart a systemic disease. Even though medicine for the past two millennia has treated cancer as purely physical, Galen (who paired it with its emotional twin of depression) understood that it was much more than a physical disturbance.

As I thought back through the four years that had turned me into a morphine-riddled, bedridden philosopher, I realized that if cancer was truly systemic, and if Galen was onto something with his careful pairing of the disease and the dis-ease, then maybe cancer was simply (simply!) the physical manifestation of a larger emotional and spiritual disturbance.

Maybe my cancer had come, at least partly, from within me.

Here I was again, physically drained after open-heart surgery, feeling powerless, and unsure of how to recover. Superficially healing my muscles and hormones, as I had attempted to do after chemo, wasn't going to be enough. Experiences and emotions flashed through my mind: My demanding professional pace. My seething anger with Michael and myself during the eight months before diagnosis. The emotional trauma of the diagnosis itself. The horrific moments of chemo. The fear that drove me into my first surgery. The frustration, desire to control, and sense of obligation that led me back to work. My fury toward my changed body. My brain's inability to do my job as I once had. Holding my breath for my fragile marriage, hoping to avoid another fallout now that the latest health crisis was seemingly behind us. My confusion and heartbreak—both literal and figurative—over where I now found myself.

If cancer really was my holistic, physical manifestation of my own dis-ease, then my recovery needed to go beyond simply killing the virulently multiplying cells. If cancer was shadow, then I needed to recognize it, acknowledge it, and strip myself bare to truly recover.

I saw the wave I'd been riding for my entire life fall away and vanish into the distance.

Well, shit, I thought as Jake tackled Ellie, returning the favor, and the two of them rolled into the hallway in an eight-legged ball of fur. *Where do I even begin?*

The next afternoon, I woke up to the phone ringing. My friend Lilly had heard about the surgery from Michael. She was shocked at how chipper I sounded.

"You are *not allowed* to sound this cheerful when your life is *this ridiculous*!" she stated before promptly bursting into tears.

"Well, to be fair," I replied, "I'm on a lot of drugs."

Lilly was raised in an enclave of wealthy privilege but yanked herself out of it in her twenties to become a social worker. Her life then unfolded in entirely unpredictable ways as she drove her Porsche to help the homeless, feeding both their bodies and their minds for her weekly *seva*, or selfless service. That morning, though, this amazing woman was on a different mission. She had called to inform me, unequivocally, that I was going to New Mexico to see her healer and sit in a sweat lodge.

"What are you talking about?" I asked. "You have a relationship with an indigenous healer? Who has that?" She made some unsympathetic noises about sticking to the point, to which I responded, "I sleep eighteen hours a day. I can barely walk because my right leg still burns every time I move. I'm not allowed to lift more than ten pounds because my chest is broken. And you're telling me that I'm about to get on a plane to New Mexico to visit a healer who I've never heard of and sit in a sweat lodge?"

Lilly was unwavering. "Yes, that's exactly what I'm telling you. You look like hell. Bring a small wheelie suitcase, wear something that shows your scar, and beg nice men to put your luggage in the overhead bin for you. Go. Heal."

Considering I had just spent the previous day wondering where to begin, these seemed like instructions that might be worth following.

THERE WERE ABOUT twelve of us in the care of the Healer who looked anywhere from a hard forty to an easy seventy, with long black hair, a warm smile, and the feeling that you're in the care of a dad—maybe not your dad, but someone's dad. Comforted and safe. Originally from the Andes and adopted into the Lakota tribe of South Dakota, he was steeped in indigenous tradition from both North and South America. We spent our mornings in discussion with the Healer and each other about what had brought each of us to ceremony. Then every afternoon, for three days in a row, we sat in the sweat lodge.

The sweat lodge is a tent-like structure built out of fallen branches and canvas. The roof of this structure came to my waist. "You crawl in on your hands and knees, offering thanks to your ancestors and Mother Earth," the Healer instructed. "Then, at the conclusion, you crawl out reborn. Oh, and crawl clockwise. And don't crawl through the hole dug in the middle."

Wedged between the Healer (who was aware of my recent physical trauma) and another woman, I shuffled along the packed dirt on my knees, my arms securely wrapped around my sternum, eventually making it around the shallow hole to land back toward the entrance.

During sweat lodge, fire-heated lava rocks are brought in, a few at a time, and placed in the shallow hole. The door drops, water is poured on the rocks, and the resulting steam instantly transported me to a space of such physical discomfort that my brain decided to leave me in the hands of the Healer and whichever of my ancestors had decided to show up and help. As in my experience with my bony pain, I found that focusing on the instant moment—the prayer being said, the smell of burning incense, the warm moisture of the steam, the gorgeous voices mingling in thousand-year-old song—allowed any discomfort to dissipate. Grace? Possibly.

After my first sweat, my five-week-old broken sternum no longer required pain medication.

After my second, my right leg no longer burned when I contracted my thigh muscles.

I wandered around, refilling my water bottle four or five times a day, with my mind quiet—none of the constant jibber-jabbering of ideas and thoughts and schemes and questions. Typically, I can quiet my mind only through meditation or sleep. That weekend, it checked itself at the entrance and let me be. That peace alone was worth the price of the plane ticket.

I cried. A lot. Most of the time, I had no idea why. And even though my mind was quiet, some of my old controlling habits persisted. The Healer made fun of me for taking notes: "Always writing, always thinking. When do you ever just be?"

One afternoon, we cooked dinner in what appeared to be a mud igloo. We had sealed the door with mud, and I found myself keeping the igloo company, slathering more mud over little cracks. The Healer's wife came over for a chat, and I jokingly said that I couldn't seem to leave the poor igloo alone.

Her response: "Of course you can't. You're immersing yourself in Mother Earth, and she's helping to heal you."

I was charmed to think Mother Earth was taking time out of her busy day of healing our endangered planet to heal little old me. I learned later that she's capable of doing both at the same time. Perhaps women get their multitasking skills from her.

On the last morning, while we were all packing to leave, I asked the Healer to help me with a dream from the previous night's sleep. "A huge black cat walked up to my sleeping bag and just looked at me," I recounted. "Jaguar, panther, I don't know. It wasn't threatening. It just stood there and looked at me. And stayed with me until I woke up."

He took a sharp intake of breath. "You need to change something. And you need to change it quickly." His response took me by surprise. He had never seemed urgent or concerned until this moment.

"Change what? What do you mean?"

The Healer paused before inviting me to go for a stroll. Then we were moved away from where anyone else could hear what he was about to say. "There are two ways we communicate with Mother Earth. We can go to her through meditation, sweat lodge, vision quests . . . any number of ways, really. Or she comes to us in our dreams."

He explained that Mother Earth had come for me, probably many times in my life before now, but most obviously a couple of years ago with cancer.

"She needs you for something," he continued. "You began to make some changes after cancer, but in your effort to fit back into your old life, you lost your focus. So she came for you again a few weeks ago. Because you're stubborn, she made this one obvious and acute. You need to pay attention to this. To her. Otherwise, the next time, she might kill you."

I took a deep breath as I balanced his words against my skepticism. My frustration with all of it—years of illness, failure of best-laid plans, inscrutability of a forward path—mounted in the face of his kind but vague counsel.

"But what am I supposed to do?" I pleaded. "It would be easier if her messages came with instructions, you know."

He smiled. "You do nothing."

"What? But you just told me I needed to make a change or she's going to smash me like a bug! This is remarkably unhelpful." I smiled back in an attempt to make my rude words less personal.

He was clearly practiced at not taking things personally. "What do you want to do? What is your heart telling you to do?"

I stopped and listened to my heartbeat for a minute. "Well, I've wanted to quit my job since returning to it after cancer. But they have been so good to me, and I have zero ideas on what I would do for money if I quit . . ." I gazed into the distance, where the violent blue sky was crashing into the orange rocks of the desert.

"I understand your conflict. But what is more important to you: your obligation to them, or your obligation to your own deep-seated desires?" His accent made the phrase *deep-seated desires* sound vitally important.

I jumped to my own conclusion: "You're telling me to quit my job."

"I'm not telling you to do anything except quiet your mind and listen to your heart." Though I watched his face intently, it gave nothing away.

Sighing, I checked back in with my breath and my heart, and found stillness. "Is this what you mean by 'do nothing'?"

His poker face broke, and he smiled. I could almost hear Yoda saying, *You are learning well, my young Padawan.*

As I stepped into the car to leave the Healer's land of vivid colors and baffling instructions, I found him at my side with his hand on the door. He seemed concerned, full of urgency, and as panicky as a spiritual wise man can be.

"Please remember to listen to your heart," he advised. "Mother Earth needs you for something, otherwise she wouldn't have come for you so urgently and at such a young age. Make whatever changes you believe will make you able to hear her more clearly. Meditate daily, just for five minutes. Listen."

I must have looked as appalled as his words made me feel.

"Yes," he nodded, "this is urgent. And yes, you need to do something, and you need to do it now. But don't panic. She won't desert you; you just need to listen. Go to her. It's less painful and much less dangerous than forcing her to come to you."

THE HEALER HAD hugged me gently and sent me home, physically pain-free and mentally in turmoil. As the number of hours that I needed to sleep ticked down from fourteen to twelve to ten—and as the number of weeks left before I was scheduled to return to work ticked down from five to four to three—I began to panic.

For thirty-plus years, I had built a life devoted to a certain version of professional success. This success required a sharp and nimble mind, a strong body to manage the long hours, a certain level of disregard for my own needs and concerns, and unfaltering devotion. Yet bolstered by the clarity of heart surgery and the force of the Healer's advice, I knew I couldn't return to the law firm.

Even so, quitting my job with no idea of what to do in its stead felt more like I was quitting my life, and that scared me to no end. I paced the house in relentless circles, not only to fulfill my clinical instructions to keep exercising my heart back to health, but also because I couldn't sit still in my own skin. I couldn't see through the fog of the past several years, so I started coming up with reasons that quitting my job was crazy.

The easiest excuse was financial, but Michael squashed that the first time I brought it up. "Once you don't need your clothing for work, we don't need your income," he said, only half joking. He made a good point: We had cats, not children. Our spending could very easily be contained.

I was scandalized by the idea. "But what kind of feminist am I if I rely on my husband's income?"

"The kind that just had cancer and heart surgery." His tone was light.

My reaction was swift and equally light. "Fuck you."

"I love you too." His eyes matched his words—he really believed that I needed to do this for myself.

I glared at him. "But what do I do then? I can't just quit!" I waved my hands violently in front of my face as if I'd just walked into a cloud of mosquitoes.

He ignored my increasing volume. "What do you want to do?" he asked calmly.

"I want to write. It's the only thing I've done since I started chemo that has helped me see things clearly. But that's not a job!"

"It *is* a job—it's just not one that provides a paycheck. Immediately . . ." He started to chuckle. "Or ever."

"This isn't funny!" My wrath was building along with the feeling that he wasn't taking me seriously. "I need to earn money!"

He smiled. "Didn't we just have that conversation?"

I stuck my tongue out at him, sank into a kitchen chair, and laid my head on the table, suddenly exhausted. I was nowhere near full-strength, either mentally or physically—whatever that now meant for me. And my physical exhaustion hit me at random moments through the day.

"I'm so tired," I complained to my elbow and the soft wooden grain under my nose.

CONVALESCENCE HAD ALWAYS struck me as a pathetic and Victorian word, implying a drooling geriatric in a wheelchair, lap covered with a blanket, glassily staring out over some green or blue vista, attended by white-hatted nurses and doting grandchildren. This image popped into my head as I sat at the kitchen table, my husband's words softly knocking on my obstreperous mind.

Perhaps, I thought in a fleeting moment of wisdom, *convalescence actually means recognizing and surrendering to the process of recovery from the true damage of illness.*

Chemo attacks every single cell in the human body. Every. Single. One. It is most efficient with fast-growing cells, but it damages all of them, in every physical part that belongs to you. Every organ. Every bone. Every muscle and tendon and ligament. Every vein and artery. Compound that with open-heart surgery, and I was a mess.

The image of drooling in a wheelchair on the shores of some lake in Switzerland suddenly seemed like not only an appealing choice, but the only one I had left.

I delayed my return to work for a week to travel with Michael to Peru. He had a speaking gig in Lima, and the company offered to take him and his wife to Machu Picchu as payment. Given my newfound love of indigenous teachings, I was going. Heart surgery and diminished lung power be damned!

I ate ceviche for two days in Lima and then spent our eighteen hours at eleven thousand feet in Cusco collapsed in bed with coca leaves and gallons of water. I napped in the van on the way to Machu Picchu, but as we drove into the Sacred Valley, something nudged me awake. And for the entirety of the time we spent in the Sacred Valley and up on Machu Picchu itself, I had more energy than I could remember having since chemo began.

I started talking to the other people on the trip—and not just talking, but nattering and cracking jokes. When we got on the train that would take us to the base of the mountain, I relentlessly paced up and down the center aisle, chatting with everyone in our little group, demanding partners for playing games, and generally behaving like a five-year-old after consuming a banana split with all the toppings, especially hot fudge and at least five cherries.

The mania immediately dissipated when I stepped through Machu Picchu's carefully maintained entrance, but the energy and strength that coursed through my wasted muscles remained. I climbed huge stairs and walked at least three miles that day. I felt buoyed and supported, rested and calm. My thoughts flickered for a moment to the spiritual power ascribed to that particular mountaintop, and I whispered a silent prayer of gratitude, just in case the power was real.

Near the end of the afternoon, as we gathered ourselves to head back down the mountain to the Sacred Valley below, Michael stopped and pointed at my legs with a horrified look on his face. I looked down. Hundreds of tiny gnats were gnawing on my skin, covering me from knees to ankles. They were so enthusiastic that blood was trickling down my legs and staining my bright green ankle socks.

"Oh, my GOD!" I shrieked. "I'm being eaten!"

One member of our little group started swatting at my legs, but I scampered out of her reach.

"No, no, no, no . . . you don't understand!" I was jumping up and down in excitement. I hadn't gotten a mosquito bite since chemo began. "I don't know what these gnats are doing, but if they find my blood delectable, then I'm going to let them have it!"

Our guide, who knew my story, stopped and looked at me. "Or," he said quietly, "maybe they're cleaning your blood for you. To help you heal."

I immediately sobered, and everyone in our small group took a step back from me, their eyes widening.

I stared at the waves of black dots on my skin and noticed for the first time that I couldn't feel the bites. I looked at Michael, who had no bugs on him. I looked at the others, who weren't being bitten either. And then I looked back at my legs. I sat down hard on a rock at my feet and burst into tears.

The group quietly moved off, each one touching my head or my shoulder as my lungs gasped for air. I sat, weeping, as the gnats drank my blood and the spirits of the mountain soothed my battered psyche.

That night, my skin showed no evidence of the voracious swarm, other than dried rivulets of blood.

As I stared at my legs, I realized that I could freak out, or I could suspend disbelief. Freaking out seemed like a waste of time and energy, so I decided to believe. I watched with fascination a few months later when the first North American mosquito since chemo landed on my arm and bit down in delight.

I whispered a prayer of gratitude to Peru as I slapped it dead.

FORWARD

FOUR DAYS AFTER returning from Peru, I was back in my office. I tried keeping the door open to welcome those who noticed my return, but I kept having to jump up and close it as waves of misery hit me. My inner type A, pantsuit-wearing high achiever had reached the point where even she was convinced that where I sat was a mistake.

My second week back, I took one of the firm's partners out to coffee and laid my internal conflict on the table between us, sniffing into my green tea and trying not to cry.

"Lydia, look at me," my friend demanded.

I slowly raised my head to peer into his kind eyes.

"To begin with, we are a billion-dollar partnership. What you have cost us, in raw dollars, is barely a blip on our balance sheet. You owe us nothing. Please understand that. You have had cancer and heart surgery. We've had associates who were less productive than you are on your worst day, who treaded water here for months before they left with no excuse other than wanting to keep earning their paycheck. If you wanted to tread water for six months or a year in order to try to regain your physical footing, not a single one of us would hold it against you."

I was surprised by his honesty.

"But if you wake up every morning feeling like your soul is being sucked out of your body, then you really shouldn't tread water here. You are too dynamic of a person to try to fit yourself back into this building if your shape no longer allows for it."

We sat quietly for a minute. And the thing that scared me the most poured out of me before I could stuff it back into my mouth.

"But I don't know what my shape is anymore," I whispered, simultaneously aghast and proud of myself for finally admitting it out loud.

"Well," he said, sipping his coffee, "you're certainly not going to figure it out by continuing to work here. This is one way of looking at one part of this world. You are very good at it. But if you don't know whether it's what you want, then you have to go and look at other parts of this world." He paused, coffee cup in midair. "If it makes you feel any better, I'll miss working with you."

Gratitude flooded through me as I considered the good fortune that this person was working at this firm with me at this point in my life. "Can I have some time to think about this?" I asked.

"Of course you can," he replied. "Take all the time you need. But please remember that your soul is more important—to me, to your colleagues, and especially to you—than this job."

Apparently, Healers come in all shapes and sizes.

WHILE I TURNED this unexpected and empowering conversation over in my head for several weeks, my health continued to occupy a tremendous amount of my time and energy. Dr. Levi still wanted me to be scanned and pricked and monitored. I had weekly appointments with Ruth and my acupuncturist, both of whom were working to help me clear the fog around my head and my body created by chemo and heart surgery. My exhaustion lay on me like a heavy sweater in summertime, and I was getting angrier and angrier about all of it. I felt like I was still moving backward.

"Oh. You have a scan on Tuesday." Michael sat in the passenger seat of our car, scrolling through his phone and schedule for the week ahead.

I was driving us home from the airport on the Sunday after Thanksgiving, four weeks after I returned to work. It had been a hilarious family weekend, and we were both tired and overfed.

"That's right. I do. And I'm glad you mentioned it."

"Do you still not want to do it?"

"Not in the slightest," I insisted.

I didn't understand why Dr. Levi wanted me to have a scan almost four months after the fluid they pulled out of my heart sac (when they poked a hole in my heart and forced me to have open-heart surgery and recover from yet another fucking sternotomy) showed that I still didn't have cancer—which I knew, and therefore the test was stupid in the first place, and if she and Michael hadn't insisted on it, then I wouldn't have had open-heart surgery, and I'd be able to run for more than a block and have a beautiful, thin, white scar instead of this monstrosity.

And I told him so as I waved in the general direction of my red, jagged, chelated cleavage.

Michael's expression came dangerously close to an eye-roll. "Your ability to look backward in order to predict the future is sometimes breathtaking."

Already frayed, I immediately bristled. "Stop being condescending, and I'm sorry to be jumping all over you, but the only thing this scan will show is that I'm fine. So I don't understand the point of going through the whole process. You're not the one who has to drink fucking barium or have a huge needle jammed into your scarred veins or sit in a goddamn tube with radiation pummeling you, which will probably give you cancer again in twenty years."

I took a deep breath that bordered on a sob. Then I slowed down to 60 mph and pulled out of the left lane. The dark Chicago night flashed by as we drove southeast toward downtown.

"I know, and I'm sorry," he answered. "I can't put myself in your position, but you really need to stop denying some very basic facts."

"Like what?" I challenged.

"You couldn't *breathe* over the summer. Which, in case you've forgotten, was one of your symptoms when you were first diagnosed. And your scan showed fluid around your heart. I can't believe you're just ignoring all that."

"I'm not ignoring it. I'm just telling you that it had nothing to do with *cancer*, so I don't want to get another *cancer* test because *I DON'T HAVE CANCER ANYMORE*." The whole disaster was caused because they'd removed the wires and bothered my heart. No matter what anyone said, that was *NOT CANCER*.

I was bordering on hysterical, desperately wanting Michael to see my perspective. Desperately wishing he would stop treating me like a perpetual cancer patient. Desperately wishing I could stop being a cancer patient.

"The thoracic surgeons said they'd never seen symptoms like that before."

"I don't care what those fucking children in the ER said. Dr. McLean admitted it was probably the wires that did it."

"Yes, but they only discovered that *after* they did the test, *after* they poked the hole in your heart, and *AFTER* Dr. Shuman opened up your chest to clean everything up and didn't see anything that might resemble cancer!"

"So what you're saying is that the goddamn CT scan *didn't* show cancer. So I don't need another scan *four months later . . .* if *EVER*." I passed a minivan going 40 mph and thought about flipping off the driver and honking. I stopped myself—not only because it was childish, but because Michael would accuse me of being childish.

"Talk to Levi." His voice sounded tired.

"She's just going to want another scan."

"You should have this conversation with her."

"It's not going to go anywhere."

We sat in silence. Usually, Michael fiddles with the radio as we drive, searching out whatever random indie band has his attention that week. But this time, he sat quietly.

I drove aggressively, fuming and upset and about to sob like a small child. I knew he was only being like this because he wanted me healthy; but at that moment, I hated him. I felt abandoned and unheard.

He took a breath and tried again. "Maybe Dr. Levi wants to have this one scan to make sure the last thing in your file shows that you're completely clean. It's a way for her to feel comfortable, like putting a period at the end of your treatment."

I immediately unbent. It was actually a really good point. I reached for Michael's hand, lying on his left thigh. He gave it to me and started stroking my thumb.

"That's a fair point," I conceded. "I'll text her tomorrow." I kept driving with my left hand on the steering wheel and my right wrapped in Michael's love—mentally scattered and physically scarred, but emotionally buoyed.

I HAD MY CT SCAN, which showed nothing of interest. Then I sought out a new, integrated doctor, with the hope that someone trained in both Western and other traditions of medicine would help me move forward and encourage my body and energy to achieve some semblance of functionality. I found Dr. Davids through desperation after my general practitioner and Dr. Levi basically ran out of advice—other than *Give it time*—on how to handle recovering from chemo.

In my very first appointment, Dr. Davids sat with me for over an hour, going over every aspect of my health history, starting with whether my mother gave birth to me naturally or through Cesarean section (the latter) and continuing through the heart surgery. For the first time in three years, cancer and chemo weren't the main topic of conversation.

Then Dr. Davids put down his pen and looked me straight in the eye. "I have terrible news for you," he stated calmly.

I slumped down in my chair. "Oh no, what? Am I dying? I didn't make the changes that the jaguar told me to change fast enough, and now Mother Earth is killing me?" Part of me felt resigned to my fate. Another part of me hoped that death would at least let me sleep. Another part of me stared, horror-struck, at the parts of me that had just given up. These despairing voices were new.

Dr. Davids laughed. "No, you're not dying. But you're not really supposed to be alive." He paused to take a breath. "You are one of the finest examples of antibiotics and modern medicine thwarting the theory of survival-of-the-fittest that I've ever seen. You should have died sometime around age three, with your first ear infection. Antibiotics saved your life, but they also did something else, which helped put you on the road to my office today." He paused again, looking at my carefully arranged expression. "They threw your genetically weak immune system entirely out of balance."

I stared at him, thunderstruck, as he explained that antibiotics kill more than the bad bacteria. They kill all the good bacteria as well, which allows other bad guys to flourish. This, in turn, taxed my immune system, which already was not qualified to keep me alive in this modern world of chemicals and pollution.

His diagnosis: a severe immune system imbalance. Starting when I was a little kid, I'd been dealing with health issues that, on the one hand, show immune system deficiencies: chronic bronchitis, annual flu, strep throat. On the other hand, there were issues that revealed overactive immune responses, such as allergies to medicines and asthma. As I had aged, my system had relinquished more and more of its balance. So instead of a mild allergic reaction to the sun and exertional asthma attacks, I had massive allergic reactions to practically every medicine I'd ever received. Instead of bronchitis, I got cancer. Then chemo damaged everything further, and now I was just exhausted from heart surgery.

It was the most logical and concise version of my health history that I had ever heard from anyone with a medical degree. I suddenly remembered that at age ten, I'd developed a nervousness about my own health, a fear that something bigger was going on that cough syrup wasn't going to cure. I had calmed myself down by becoming an athlete, ensuring that I would stay physically strong.

"We need to bring you back into balance," Dr. Davids announced. "We'll start with your gut flora, because they are the center of everything. This should help balance your hormones, because your endocrine system is wrapped around your digestive system. After that, we'll go where your symptoms lead us." He started writing out a list of foods to avoid because they would burden my system (gluten, dairy, alcohol) and a list of supplements that I needed to start taking (too many, with high-powered probiotics first on the list).

"But I'm pretty sure my hormones are back on track," I protested. "I mean, my period shows up once every fourteen to forty days."

"That just means your hormones are present. A cycle that irregular is not on track." He told me to think of my hormone system like a waterfall, with the thymus and the adrenals at the top. "If they are working properly, then we go to the thyroid, and we move on from there. The sex hormones are actually at the bottom of this list. Once we sort out the top of the waterfall, your period and sex hormones should regulate on their own."

I chewed on this piece of information, frustrated that this was the first time I'd heard of my endocrine system in such a logical way. At the thought of my missing thymus, which should be at the top of this waterfall, I swallowed a flash of anger at Levi and McLean.

"We need to trick your body into thinking that you still have your thymus," Dr. Davids continued, explaining about blood tests, DHEA, and how we would work our way down the waterfall. "Only once we've gotten everything else on track will we worry about your sex hormones. Or—and this would be ideal—they'll just regulate themselves once everything above them works properly again." He paused. "Do you want children anytime soon?"

Ah, my favorite question. "I have no idea if I want them at all, but I certainly don't want them while I'm feeling like this. It's just that my period was an obvious symptom that something is wrong."

He smiled. "It is a symptom of that, absolutely. I'm glad you came in. Working together, we can alleviate your exhaustion and finally regulate your period. But it's not going to happen overnight. It has taken a long time to get your body this out of balance—it's going to take a long time and a lot of effort to get it back into balance."

The constant refrain of *Give it time* was still annoying, but at least he had coupled it with a cohesive and understandable plan toward health. This gave my exhausted mind a small thrill.

"Oh, I do need you to do something in addition to the protocol of supplements and dietary changes." Dr. Davids threw this comment out as though it were an afterthought.

"What's that?" I shrugged my jacket on, checking my pockets. *Wallet, keys, phone . . .*

"Meditate for at least an hour a day. You're unbelievably stressed, and you're revving too high as a result. You need to meditate to bring your adrenals and thyroid back down to earth."

I stopped and stared at him. "Seriously? You're an MD, and you're prescribing meditation?"

"Yes, and your blood work will tell me if you're not doing it. Also, you are working as a corporate lawyer?"

"Yes." I was suddenly wary of the direction this conversation was going.

"Can you quit?"

I bowed my head in acknowledgment but didn't say anything. I was finally beginning to recognize that perhaps this was what the Healer had meant by his instruction.

Listen.

There wasn't a massive conspiracy between Dr. Davids and the partner at work and my teacher from New Mexico. This was advice coming at me, independently, from all sorts of directions. Perhaps I should start to listen. And maybe, just maybe, to act.

I wondered how much of my life I had spent fighting these kinds of messages, and I decided right then that this was a habit I absolutely had to break.

The next day, five weeks after I returned to work from heart surgery, I gave my notice at the law firm. They weren't surprised, and all of them, without exception, completely understood. One even asked if I needed extra money to help me through the transition.

I TOLD THE OFFICE that I was quitting to write a book about my experience. Of course, I had no concrete plans to do so. Despite all the messages and conversations, I still couldn't just say, *I quit because I need to recover!* I had to appease the part of my personality that needed a goal.

I was still going to my therapy appointments, but writing was the only thing that could really pull me through my emotional fog. My hazy memories. My fear of being a perpetual patient. My fury with my doctors. My gratitude toward my doctors. My changed relationship with my husband and friends and family.

Writing had helped me get through chemo with some semblance of sanity and a sense of humor, but I had been so tired and muddled in the subsequent months that it had fallen by the wayside. It wasn't just that I hadn't been posting to my blog. I hadn't been writing at all.

The part of me that still basked in the New Mexico sun knew this wasn't just a mistake. It was dangerous. Now that I had the time and could force myself to start writing again, I might finally start to see through the fog.

I walked out of the office for the last time on January 2, 2015. I stepped into the brutality of winter in Chicago—the wind off the lake, heavy and wet, ripping through clothing on a mission to freeze bones. Everything grey, unless there were sunny blue skies heralding temperatures well below zero. I walked away from a life that I had sprinted toward for more than thirty years. Fancy university, political job, five years of graduate school completed in three, marriage, fancy law job, followed by deterioration of marriage, cancer, chemo, and striving to get back to work, get back to life, get back to *NORMAL*—followed by heart surgery.

Is there a word faster than *sprint*?

My version of academic success had translated into powerful professional success in the corporate and political world. And I walked away from it . . . why? Because a Healer and a big black cat had told me to? Because my "gut" had been screaming about it? Because of a doctor's mistake too close to my heart?

Yup.

My professional success, in the wake of everything that had happened to me, didn't even look like success anymore. It looked like all the reasons that I had gotten cancer and that my marriage had hit such a huge speed bump.

After nearly dying during heart surgery, I finally knew that I couldn't go back. After everything that had happened, I didn't even want to go back. But that didn't stop fear from creeping in around the edges. I was changing everything about how I had always lived my life, and even though I knew it was the best thing for me, I was scared shitless.

The city layered its winter on top of my fear and drove me to hibernation. I've always detested Chicago's winter. As it wrapped me in its frigid, ugly embrace, the reasons I changed my life started to drift away. It all seemed so stupid.

I sank, deeply and powerfully, into cancer's emotional twin —the dis-ease of depression.

MICHAEL AND LILLY (Sweat Lodge-Lilly, as Elizabeth calls her) gave me exactly two weeks of being unable to move from the couch for something other than bourbon or red wine or a bathroom break. Then they frog-marched me (metaphorically) to

Lilly's house in Florida. She dumped me on the beach for a week, took me out to dinners and movies, and reminded me that she was a social worker and was now officially part of the team that was putting Humpty Dumpty back together again. Above all, she wrapped me in enough love and sunshine to loosen the stranglehold of fear and doubt.

Next, I went to my childhood home in Washington, DC, to help my parents with the kind of projects that only happen after spending thirty years in the same house—basement and garage inventory and cleanup—which made me feel useful again. The tasks were big enough to keep me focused for a few months. What Lilly had started, combined with the pride and delight of being helpful to my parents, fully snapped me out of my melancholy. My father came to visit me in Chicago in March and returned the favor, helping me clean up the room where I would spend my time writing. And at last, I began this new, completely foreign stage of my life.

I took my dad with me for company when I went back to Dr. Davids for my first follow-up. I had quit my job, meditated, donated my blood to dozens of tubes, peed into a sterile cup, undergone a stool test, and spit into various vials in the interim. One of the results pointed to heavy metal toxicity, and we needed to update the plan.

"I feel like I'm just playing Whack-A-Mole," I complained. "I've been meditating and taking supplements, and I even quit my damn job, but I'm still exhausted. And now I have massive doses of barium, lead, and mercury in my system." I was collapsed in a chair, slumped so far down that I was practically sitting on my own neck. From my posture to my voice, I was walking defeat.

Dr. Davids ignored my pessimism. “Instead of Whack-A-Mole, can we think of your health as peeling away the layers of an onion?”

In order to get as sick as I got, he explained, I had started out with a little problem that then got bigger and bigger and bigger until it turned into cancer. Cancer was the outer layer of the onion. Cancer treatment added a few more layers on top—things like fertility and various hormone imbalances, a shell-shocked and depleted immune system, and general fatigue. I’d been peeling away the layers ever since I stopped chemo, mostly by sleeping a lot. But my endocrine and immune systems were still beleaguered. After all, they’d been out of balance for over thirty years.

“As I told you before,” he continued, “it’s going to take more than a few months to reset. And every time we discover the reason behind some of your symptoms, it gives us another way to support you back to health. This is good news!”

I went home with a prescription for chelating agents that would start pulling the metals out of my system. Then I spent a few hours writing and took a nap with Ellie while my father read with Jake splayed out next to him, feet in the air. Baby steps forward.

A FEW MONTHS later, my acupuncturist pulled out a needle from my leg, leaned over the puncture site, and said, “Well, that’s interesting.”

I spend my acupuncture appointments napping on my back on the table, and it usually takes a solid couple of hours to feel fully awake afterward. At her words, though, I sat up and leaned back on my elbows, immediately present. "What's interesting? You know I don't like being interesting."

She chuckled while still leaning over my shins. "Well, a little trickle of water just came out of the needle hole."

"WHAT?" I sat bolt upright on the treatment table to look at my leaking shin. The acupuncturist wasn't kidding—a small drop of water was making its way down the side of my calf.

She stayed clinical. "Have you been swollen recently?"

"Yes." As proof, I waved my fingers at her and attempted to remove my wedding band.

"How long?"

I laughed. This had not been my main focal point. "I have no idea. Probably since I gained back all the weight I lost during chemo, and then some. So, I don't know, two years? I just assumed it would go away with exercise."

She smiled. "Apparently not."

I reported this to Dr. Davids.

"Well," he said, waving a test result in the air, "that makes sense."

I glared at him. "*Now* what?"

"You have a massive yeast colony living in your gut."

"Awesome."

The gut is a delicately balanced ecosystem of thousands of species of bacteria, some yeast, and even some viruses and parasites. They are all supposed to stay inside the ecosystem and duke it out amongst themselves. Good bacteria keeps it all in check while working with digestive enzymes from the liver to fully digest food. In a healthy gut, the balance is supposed to be about 80 percent good bacteria to 20 percent everything else.

When a person takes full-spectrum antibiotics, all the bacteria are killed off, both good and bad, so the bad guys flourish. This is made worse by the American diet full of sugar and carbs, which bad bacteria and yeast love to eat, and when an immune system is compromised because of illness. AIDS, cancer, and organ transplant patients are all susceptible to gut chaos and associated illness.

Yeast is supposed to stay in the gut, but when the gut is plagued by yeast and bad bacteria, it starts seeping into the bloodstream. This causes chaos for the immune system fighters, which are focused on battling everything else in our environment—they aren't designed to fight yeast in the blood. If the immune system is already compromised through illness, the body simply can't handle the new intruder. Then yeast takes up residence outside of the gut causing—ahem—chronic fatigue, lack of energy, low libido, fuzzy brain, irritability, cramping, bloating, unpleasantness in the gastrointestinal tract, vaginal and urinary yeast infections, bladder infections, irritable bladder, food sensitivity, allergies, eczema, and sugar cravings, to name but a few ailments.

As Dr. Davids said, we were continuing to peel back the onion.

My ratio was the opposite of normal: 80 percent bad to 20 percent good. The bad was evenly divided between yeast and bad bacteria. In other words, my gut was a disaster.

Within two weeks of starting the extremely regimented three-month treatment for the yeast (which included a prescription and eating zero sugar, added or natural, and zero carbs), my edema went away. Ten pounds simply melted off my body.

With all this medical stuff happening at the pace of onion peeling, I realized that in order to live through it with any semblance of patience, I was going to have to completely relaunch my own relationship with my body. I was beyond furious and frustrated with my body, completely fed up with its excuses—cancer, heart surgery, yeast, enough! But it was the only one that was going to get me through the rest of my life.

Before I could forgive my body, I needed to recognize the full extent of my anger toward it. So out it poured, into my journal.

I described how my always strong, supple, athletic, sexual, beautiful body had just stopped working the way I knew it to work, and how my self-confidence shattered along with it. I wrote about how chemo stripped me of my physical beauty . . . and how I had to learn, on a deep inner level, what true strength and beauty were . . . and how annoying and exhausting it was to keep reminding myself that even emaciated and bald, with no eyelashes and no energy, I was still strong and beautiful.

I put it all down on paper—how when I gained my weight back, I had no energy and couldn't do anything with my new weak, flabby body. Sex was nonexistent for months, and then it hurt. Then my beautiful husband and I had to sort through the fact that I had almost died on him more times than a man in his thirties should have to expect. The whole thing made me angry and confused, which then made me feel like my brain and spirit were somehow damaged too. And it had all started with my body's failure to return magically to the body that I once knew.

As I wrote, I realized that if my body had betrayed my idealized expectations of it, it was really only returning the favor. For years, I had been asking it to do more for me than any sane person would demand: Stay in shape even though my workouts were sporadic. Stay slender even though I drank alcohol, ate food that wasn't always healthy, and lived among cars and breathed God-knows-what toxins. Stay calm even though my life was one big stress test. I had betrayed my body just as much as it had betrayed me.

And I wondered why it had given up?

I sat and wrote, and I stared out my window, vacillating between sadness and anger as this realization sank in. Then I noticed my recently acquired tattoo: Sanskrit words that meant "Peaceful, Grounded, Strength." Because it was done in white ink on my inner left arm, it looked like a faded scar, which generally meant I was the only one who could see it. That's why I had it done that way. It was not for public consumption. But I wanted the message somewhere I could see it as often as possible.

Those words had come to me in my mid-twenties during a particularly difficult yoga class. They had stayed with me ever since, and I relied on them whenever I felt like I had little control: staying still during a CT scan, breathing through a tough conversation, holding a yoga pose that was asking too much of me. In many respects, they acted as a meditation mantra. They were so helpful during chemotherapy that I wanted to keep them with me permanently. Hence the tattoo.

I stared at the tattoo, noticing that a real scar now ran through it—a thin scratch from Jake, about three inches long. It moved with my arm as I flipped my palm up and down. Like a creepy painting, it seemed to stare back at me.

Looking at it for a long time brought the image of a calm ocean into my head. By definition, the ocean is connected to the earth and gets its strength from that connection . . . *Grounded*. If needed, it will beat the shit out of you, but otherwise it's calm, nurturing . . . *Peaceful*. Maybe it's because I spent my childhood summers swimming in the Atlantic Ocean, but I find few things more nurturing than an ocean. The sound, the smell, the feeling of the water and sand. The fact that it can destroy so easily is part of its appeal . . . *Strength*.

Whenever I've spent an afternoon in the water, it feels as though I've done so with permission. Permission that can be revoked if I don't stay in the flow of the currents of my own life. At any given moment, the ocean can turn from a gentle, supportive float in the water to a smackdown, and suddenly I'm upside-down with a mouthful of sand, gasping for breath as the next wave crashes over me.

As I stared at my tattoo and the ocean filled my mind, I realized something: perhaps this is what patience is about. A calm ocean is patient. It is peaceful and grounded and strong. My body had been asking me to be patient with it for more than fifteen years, ever since those words dropped into my mind, and I had been ignoring it.

This was the beginning of a full-on meltdown, so I called Ruth.

"But if my body has been asking for patience," I entreated, "why didn't it drop the word *patience* into my mind all those years ago?"

"Because you wouldn't have listened," Ruth responded. "For you, patience is a dirty word. Think about how much you were trying to achieve in such a short amount of time. You needed to hear the message differently."

I looked at my arm again.

Peaceful
Grounded
Strength

"So all this time, I've been asking myself to be patient."

She deflected my self-judgment before I let it take hold. "No. You've been asking yourself, and striving, to be peaceful and grounded and strong. Some days you achieved one or two. Sometimes you would achieve all three. What did it feel like on the days when you achieved all three?"

I looked back over my life, and memories of those days flickered before me: Calming my sister during her first chemo treatment, as she tried to rip the IV out of her arm and jump out the window. Sitting in Hero Pose on the floor in my hospital room, welcoming the sensation as tightness drained from my thighs. Taking the bar exam, both feet planted firmly on the ground. Cuddling the kittens when they were so tiny, and I was so exhausted from the fear that they were simply going to die in my hands. Achieving that smooth feeling at around mile five of my favorite six-mile loop in Boston, long before anyone got sick.

"Pretty amazing," I admitted. "It didn't really matter what I was doing, but I was supportive and loving and calm and focused, for either myself or someone else."

"Mmm-hmmm." I could almost see Ruth nodding on the other end of the phone. "Patience doesn't sound so bad now, does it?"

ABOUT TEN MONTHS after I quit my job, seven months after I started writing this book, and exactly two weeks after Dr. Davids allowed me to start eating a limited amount of carbs again, I looked at Michael and said, with butterflies bashing around in my stomach, "So it turns out I'm nervous about two things."

We were sitting at a shitty Mexican restaurant in Idaho, and I had finally discovered what had been causing my most recent bout of writer's block. Shitty Mexican is our favorite kind of Mexican food—it's your basic meat, cheese, beans, and guacamole, wrapped up in some kind of tortilla in any number of different ways. Shitty Mexican is one of God's great comfort foods, and sometimes—as in this case, after getting up at 4 a.m. when neither of us wanted to travel, in order to catch two planes and drive for an hour to a tiny town in the middle of beautiful nowhere to celebrate a friend's wedding—it's necessary.

"Oh?" Michael slowly chewed on a tortilla chip and then took a sip of water. "What's that?"

I focused on my breathing. "You know I've been writing about us before cancer, right?"

He nodded.

"Well, I'm afraid that if I write about the time when our marriage was falling apart, it will rip apart the stitches holding our marriage together, and it's all going to happen all over again."

He nodded again. "And the other problem?" His hand moved back to the chip basket.

"I'm also a little jammed by telling someone else's story as part of my own. Specifically yours."

He picked up a chip, dipped it in salsa, and popped it in his mouth. "What makes you think that reliving the year before diagnosis will harm us?"

I paused, trying to gather the facts that had made the emotions so poignant before I laid them out in words and began the process of letting them go. "Often, when I tell aspects of the story, they completely diverge from your version. I mean, I get that we have our own versions of what happened, but if they are as different as they sometimes seem to be, then that's problematic."

He chuckled. "Obviously, we have different views of what happened. For a long time, our perspectives of the leadup to your heart surgery differed dramatically, with you blaming me and Dr. Levi for bullying you into doing the test that caused the whole disaster. Time and your own work has healed some of that, but I have a feeling we'll never be on the same page about it."

"True."

"So we have different stories around the same facts. We may even have different facts. Which, by the way, makes this your story, and not mine."

"Yeah, that's where I got with this as well."

"If, *once you have written it down*"—he gave me the stern look he reserves for when I'm not doing the work I set out to do, and he knows I'm only going to end up disappointing myself—"our versions diverge completely, then we'll talk about it. But I don't see them diverging so ridiculously that it will be anything more than a 'Let's talk about this' conversation, instead of a . . ." He drifted off.

I made the motion of someone flipping over a table in fury.

"Right," he continued. "That. And even if our stories do

diverge so ridiculously, I still don't think it will break us. I think we've moved past it."

I sifted through the emotions that popped up in response to his words. Relief. Joy. Contentment. I built a fajita—spread guacamole on the corn tortilla, add steak and onions, sprinkle cheese so it melts, spoon black beans, wrap—and started chewing.

"Would you do it again?" I asked.

"Probably."

"Would you do it again, knowing what you know now?"

"You mean, would I do the second campaign again, knowing how eviscerating it would be emotionally? Probably." He paused for a minute. "Although, if I knew you were going to get sick, I don't know that I would do it again. The combination of the two almost killed me." He said it quietly, more to his plate than to me.

I reached across the table and gently brushed the back of his hand. "If we believe that cancer is caused by some kind of stressor or emotion, I wonder if I would have gotten sick if you hadn't done the campaign. Or if I hadn't reacted to it the way I did."

"I know that you think about that a lot." He paused, blinking away emotion. "But cancer takes a long time to grow. And you were physically really strong, so it probably took longer than usual with you."

I frowned. "Dr. Levi said my tumor probably started growing about eight months before diagnosis."

"But in one way you think about this, it would have manifested as a cancerous disturbance in your energetic field a long time before it got bad enough to manifest in you physically."

"True."

We both paused to eat more comfort.

"I've been thinking about this, actually," he continued. "We joke about the ridiculous coincidences of where we were when you were diagnosed. If Mother Earth really did give you cancer in order to bring you back or put you on your right path, she may have been working a long time prior to that. She may have given you me to help you through it."

"Wait, what?" I asked, surprised at the path his thoughts had taken. Although he had witnessed and supported my emotional transformation at the hands of my indigenous healer, he didn't talk about it much.

"Think about it," he went on. "I studied immunology at NIH the summer I was nineteen and never did anything with it. I could have played lacrosse when I was a kid, but I didn't—I played soccer with the guy who ended up running Livestrong. I'm calm in a crisis. I remember everything. I went through my own shit, so I know what it takes to get through a personal war. With no disrespect to the other relationships you've had, out of all of them, I am uniquely set up to help you through a cancer diagnosis and treatment."

"Huh." I sat on that for a minute, musing. "If we take this as true, then I've been off my path for a long time." I paused, mentally sifting through my résumé to figure out where I might have gone left when I "should" have gone right.

Michael wasn't finished. "You got into one law school, and it happened to be in the city where I was living. We lived four blocks from the hospital. You switched to the law firm's amazing health insurance plan six months before you were diagnosed.

You pushed us to sign up for life insurance three months before you were diagnosed. I moved back into the apartment and our marriage the night before you were diagnosed, which proved to you that I stayed with you because I wanted to be with you, not because I felt guilty that you were sick."

I sat back. This was a little more than I was willing to handle on four hours of sleep and five hours of breathing canned airplane air.

"If we take these coincidences to their logical extreme, you were *supposed* to get cancer in 2012, and you were *supposed* to get it with me." After this remarkable inventory, he calmly ate another chip.

"So where did I go wrong?" I thought out loud.

"Maybe you didn't. Maybe you were supposed to get sick in order to give you the freedom to let go of control. In order to force you into a different way of thinking about life. In order to give you these experiences. Maybe getting sick in your thirties was simply the best way to get you where you need to be in order to do what you are supposed to do. And I was part of that. In the same way that you are here to help me get through my own landmines, I was brought into your life to help you get through yours."

He stopped for another bite of enchilada.

"And therefore, of course, your writing about all of this won't break us. Because it's part of why we're together."

I sat back, amazed. "I love you."

"As I love you."

In that moment, as in so many moments of my life, those were the only words I needed.

CHANGE

EPILOGUE

TODAY I WOKE UP, drank my usual breakfast smoothie, took a handful of supplements, and tumbled back into bed with terrible nausea. Two hours later, I had a hot flash—the first since my period returned five years ago.

Menopause. At age thirty-nine.

As the consuming heat radiated from behind my neck into the rest of my body, two thoughts flashed through my mind.

First: *Ugh.*

And then: *Finally.*

That second thought can be further divided into two parts. Michael and I have decided, with the help of time, therapy, and clear-eyed honesty—as well as a lot of eye-opening moments with human beings under the age of five and their parents—that we don't want children of our own. At the same time, I have also discovered that my new body cannot handle the toxic load of hormonal birth control. So, *Finally* part one is a response to the fact that condoms are annoying, and I'm looking forward to not using them sooner rather than later.

Finally part two is because I am excited to leave my time as a "maiden" behind me and officially graduate to "crone." The hormonal flood that women experience every month is legitimate. The by-products of this monthly flood—mood fluctuations, body changes—become second nature for us to manage, but this takes energy and focus. And I have better things to do with my energy and focus.

I have writing and learning and exploring and thinking to do. Doing all of that through an irrationally angry or weepy day is something I am capable of—because I'm capable of a lot of things. But, wow! Won't life be awesome when the energy I have always spent managing my monthly moods can be deployed elsewhere?

Plus, many cultures consider a woman to be an "elder" once menopause is complete—and that's just a cool title.

Once I stopped sweating and realized that I was no longer nauseous, I took my news to Michael, who said, "I'm sorry about the hot flashes, but am I supposed to be surprised?"

"Yes, dear, because I'm now perimenopausal, and I wasn't before." I mean, was he an idiot?

"Um, you sure?" he replied. "I'm fairly certain that you've been perimenopausal since chemo. I mean, your period has been completely irregular for a long time, and it's only gotten worse."

And then my brain exploded.

He was right. Since my period had returned five years earlier, I'd been getting it once every ten to sixty days, and those wonky intervals had become even more ridiculous over the past year. This was an integral point, and I hadn't even noticed it.

I hadn't been following my own advice.

A long while back, I had made peace with the fact that my body would never again be what it was *before*. That my mind would not be what it was *before*. That my life would not be what it was *before*. Yet I had been longing for my period to normalize and for my hormones to regulate my body as they did before I got sick.

Once again, the universe was yelling until I finally listened: *No, Lydia! You need to remember that "back" isn't a place you can go! Nothing will be the same as it was—including hormones!*

Well, shit.

Humans are not the best at managing change, so we fight it. When something in our life changes, our default move is to get things back to normal. The need to find our "normal" doesn't consider whether *back* is a place that is good or bad for us, whether going *back* is ideal or not, or even whether it is physically, mentally, emotionally, or spiritually possible to go *back*. The urge is simply to return to what we know: back to control . . . back to where we had practice being ourselves . . . back to what was comfortable, if only because it was known and familiar.

In the case of recovering from disease, in Western culture, the instruction to *go back* is often the only message we hear, whether from doctors, colleagues, fellow survivors, gym trainers, or (especially) our own inner voice. That effort to *go back* to my old body, my honeymoon marriage, my job, my life—it was a tremendous struggle. And I discovered after heart surgery that I wasn't going to find health inside that struggle.

As I eventually found out, moving forward required me to learn two things: First, that I could control only my own decisions and behavior, not the world around me. And second, that if I have a little faith (in God, Allah, the Universe-with-a-capital-*U*—whatever works, really), I'll be okay.

I believe that life, in some respects, is an exercise in accepting that I'm the only one I can actually control. And if I'm the only one I can control, then my job isn't to manage the universe or my fellow creatures. Instead, it's to learn how to manage myself with some level of grace and kindness inside the unexpected. Because whether the unexpected is welcome or not, it will happen.

The title of this book—*Wait, It Gets Worse*—started as a joke: *Oh, you thought cancer was the worst I went through? Just you wait . . .* But now, it's also my own little reminder that life is a roller coaster, so why pine for quiet or "normal"? How boring! Life won't be any of that, anyway. So if I'm waiting for the world to slow down so I can jump off (even for just a minute), I'm only setting myself up for disappointment.

Putting my health aside for a minute, the absolute worst part about recovering from my hospital visits was realizing that in order to thrive, I could no longer pretend I had control over the circumstances that surround my life. This horrible epiphany was coupled with an extraordinary one: I can, and must, control the internal. My attention. My reactions. My perspective. These are the only things I can control.

For example, I can't control Michael's choices and behavior. But I can control how I respond: with kindness or with frustration, with patience or with intolerance. All these are choices I can make around my own behavior.

I'm never going to win if I'm battling the world. Accepting this reality has brought me a great deal of peace. Now my job is to take all the wonderful bits and pieces that make up *me*—my experiences, my quick mind, my strong body, my sometimes-unfortunate personality—and encourage them all to work in harmony with each other. With that internal harmony, I approach the things I'd like to change with a much more flexible perspective.

The second aspect of moving forward instead of looking backward is both the simplest and the hardest thing of all: I have to trust that everything is going to be fine.

I know that sounds naïve and blindly optimistic, but trust me: my eyes are open, and I see what's happening. So come with me for a moment. I'm not saying that faith has taught me everything is going to unfold exactly as I'd like. If that were the case, faith would be teaching all eight billion of us that the future will unfold in eight billion ways. I'm saying the opposite: faith has taught me that things are going to unfold exactly as they are meant to unfold, and my job is to be hyperaware of what is happening, to adapt to the circumstances, and to respond in the kindest and most effective way possible. This free fall always has a soft landing, even if there are some hard bounces along the way.

I sometimes wonder what precancer Lydia would think of me now. She was loyal and dedicated, beautiful and judgey, controlling and sarcastic and complex in all the wonderful ways that made her human. Although she's not my proudest creation, she is a part of me and I love her nonetheless. But I'm also thrilled that aspects of her have shifted and now I'm the one sitting in her old body. So much of my life has spun out in ways I could have never predicted. If I had continued trying to control things, without any kind of faith that it would all be okay, I would have completely lost my mind.

My control freak still lives, but she has a different job now. She's not in charge of choosing when to activate (it used to be all the time) and what issues to regulate (it used to be everything). When something frightens me or causes anxiety, instead of trying to change the outside world, she takes a breath and waits for my brain to help me figure out what exactly is causing my agitation. Once that's sorted, she activates with strategy and plans and itineraries.

And yet obviously, regarding the change in my hormones, I had missed the boat on all that. Rather than follow my new, postcancer advice, I had instinctively hung on to the idea of *going back*. A few months of menstrual irregularity? Sure, that's easy to overlook. But five years? *Come on, Lydia*, says my newly compartmentalized control freak. *Now you're just being stubborn and willfully ignorant.*

So, what, dear brain, was holding me back? What is my internal anxiety about menopause?

Aging. Death. Loss of a toned body. A dry vagina.

Okay. Now that all my fears are laid out in front of me, my control freak can manage the fallout: Find medications in Colorado and California to manage the dryness issue. Determine exercise that I enjoy and can continue to do with an aging, post-chemo body. Take my ass to a therapist to discuss my fear of death (which, it turns out, probably isn't really the problem—but that's a story for another day). The trick to keeping the control freak in her lane is to pull my anxieties out into the open so she can do what she does best: analyze and destroy!

Sometimes it's a struggle, but I just have to constantly remember: My life will never be the same as it was before. And I don't actually want it to be (most of the time), despite the siren pull to *go back*.

Living in the present is hard, and I don't pretend that I'm remotely good at this. Having the focus to hold on to my faith, point my attention to my own behavior, and keep my control freak tasked on her job takes practice and patience. Yes, there it is again: *Peaceful. Grounded. Strength*. It is an unfinished process.

I don't spend all of my time meditating on a mountaintop somewhere, so I do mess up—and I will continue to do so. Yes, I still shout at the rain. Yes, I screw up and yell at Michael. Yes, I get mad at my body. Yes, I forget to meditate and forget to keep the faith.

What do I do when that happens? I admit it, clean it up, forgive myself, and keep going. And then do it again. And again.

As I was putting the finishing touches on this book, Michael and I received some family news that led us to return once more to the path of Huge Life Change. We put our house in Chicago on the market and began plans to transplant our lives to a quiet town on the Hudson River in New York. Three years ago, my control freak would have been managing my behavior and trying to minimize change, to keep things "normal" and comfortable. And what would be the result? I'd want to avoid the upheaval because it would be "too much." Not too much to handle—I've got broad shoulders, so I can handle a lot—but too much out of my own control. If I lived near my family, how would I keep control of my own life? How would I control their lives? How would I make all of it fit into the little box where I lived my world? In the end, we would've stayed in Chicago.

Now, a small part of me is gnashing her teeth at the fact that

I have to move (*Ugh, moving!*), learn a new grocery store layout, and figure out which shop owners are kind enough to let you use their bathroom in a pinch.

A larger part of me is desperately sad that I'm leaving my extraordinary friends, so I cry in those moments and have already started making plans to come back and visit them in Chicago.

But the largest part of me is like a kid on Christmas Eve. I have very little idea of what my life will look like next week—where I will live, or what I will do for paid employment. Yet I'm really excited to discover what's in store for me.

At the very least, I will be a more active presence in the lives of the people I love most in the world. That gift alone is worth the price.

At the most? Who knows! But I have faith that it will be incredible. Rather than letting fear keep me looking back toward what I already know, I'm trying to let the joy of my new future guide my present. That faith in the promise of my future—that joy in its possibility—grounds me more than my control freak ever did.

ACKNOWLEDGMENTS

I RARELY READ this section in books, but as I wrote my story, I realized that it exists to drag into the sunlight the real people in my life without whom this book would be an unborn child. And I will never ignore it again.

To avoid hurting the living or distressing the dead (thank you, Nabokov), I have changed many of the proper names in this story. Elizabeth, Gene, and Ruth are all composite characters, so if you recognize parts of yourself or your own story in those characters, it's because you're there. Everyone named or unnamed, in a previous manuscript or the final book, is there because you helped me live and learn and thrive.

Life is not an individual sport. Neither, despite it's solitary reputation, is writing. Although I wrote the book mostly in the company of my cats, getting my brain out of the way so that I could deliver this message took the effort of many: Sara, Madeline, Jennifer, Hernan, Marilyn, Liz, Elyshia, Ajay, Cheryl, Lizzi, Charlie, Kim, Anthony, Ashley, and everyone I've forgotten because you did such a good job of shutting down my mind.

Getting the book to production took the effort of even more: Maureen Batty, Corey Blake, Rachel Gostenhofer, and the entire magnificent team at Disruption Books, especially my extraordinarily patient and kind and brilliant editor, Kris Pauls.

To my personal squadron of soul sisters and brothers: The tears that I have dropped onto your shoulders, your appetizer plates, and cocktails helped to soothe and focus my ragged, aimless desire to simply be of use.

To my parents: You somehow managed to raise me to be headstrong and confident, love me, and keep your sanity at the same time. For that, I salute you.

To Michael, Corinna, and Ellen: Blue ribbons and gold stars and my first-born child. Seriously. All the blue ribbons and all the gold stars and all the babies.

My gratitude to each of you is boundless. Thank you, from the bottom of my scarred but thriving heart.

ABOUT THE AUTHOR

LYDIA SLABY is an advocate, speaker, and writer focused on empowering people, communities, and organizations faced with daunting change. She is an advisor to Chicago's 2nd Story, serves on the board of I AM THAT GIRL, an organization that helps young women around the world take ownership of their self-worth, and was a board member of Critical Mass: The Young Adult Cancer Alliance. She lives with her husband Michael Slaby and their two beautiful cats in Rhinebeck, New York.